BILLION DOLLAR BABY

Paul Cullen is a journalist and the author of four previous non-fiction books. Born in London, he grew up in Dublin, where he studied engineering in Trinity College Dublin. He lived in Switzerland for five years before returning to Ireland to study journalism at Dublin City University. Appointed to *The Irish Times* in 1993, he reported on health, politics, consumer affairs, international development and education in a career spanning three decades.

He wrote the bestselling book *With a Little Help from My Friends* about the planning tribunal's investigations into corruption. His memoir, *Outsider*, published in 2026, recounts how a near-fatal accident drove him to uncover long-hidden secrets about his origins. He has won many awards for his work, including Irish news journalist of the year in 2023. He lives in Dublin.

ALSO BY PAUL CULLEN

Outsider: Survival, Family Secrets and the Search to Belong
With a Little Help from My Friends: Planning Corruption in Ireland
Refugees and Asylum-Seekers in Ireland
Insight Guide to Dublin, Wicklow and the Boyne Valley

BILLION DOLLAR BABY

How Ireland Built Its National Children's Hospital – At Any Cost

PAUL CULLEN

HACHETTE
BOOKS
IRELAND

First published in Ireland in 2026 by HACHETTE BOOKS IRELAND

With thanks to the following for permission to include material in this book: *The Irish Times*, Stephen Collins (author of *The Power Game*), Leo Varadkar (author of *Speaking My Mind*) and Barry Kennerk (author of *Temple Street Children's Hospital: An Illustrated History*).

Cataloguing in Publication Data is available from the British Library.

ISBN 9781399755894

Typeset in Garamond Premier Pro by Bookends Publishing Services, Dublin

Hachette Books Ireland
8 Castlecourt Centre
Castleknock
Dublin 15, Ireland
(info@hbgi.ie)

Authorised representative in the EEA

A division of Hachette UK Ltd
Carmelite House, 50 Victoria Embankment, London EC4Y 0DZ

www.hachettebooksireland.ie

To my family

Contents

Author's Note

This account draws on scores of interviews with people involved with or affected by the children's hospital project, and on the reporting of journalists, including myself, at the time events occurred. To distinguish between these forms of source material, I use the past tense ('she said') when I am relying on the historical record and the present tense ('she says') in relation to interviews.

Hospitals in Ireland are forever changing names. The tendency is often towards longer and more unwieldy names. For a while there was a vogue for inserting the word 'university' into the title of every hospital, as if this would of itself improve the services being offered.

All this could serve to confuse the reader. Crumlin hospital started life as Our Lady's Hospital for Sick Children; Tallaght hospital as the Adelaide and Meath Hospital, Dublin, incorporating the National Children's Hospital (AMNCH); Temple Street's most recent moniker was the awkward CHI at Temple Street.

Consequently, I have adopted a broad-brushstroke approach to the hospitals referred to in the text, usually opting for the simplest form of their names.

Similarly, and again for purposes of simplification, I generally refer to the National Paediatric Hospital Development Board, the body charged with building the children's hospital, as the 'development board' or simply the 'board'. I have also, on occasion, simplified the titles of government departments to the most relevant competencies, referring for example to the 'department of public expenditure' rather than the more unwieldy 'department of public expenditure and reform'. And while BAM, the main contractor, operates through a number of companies in Ireland, I refer to it in the text simply as 'BAM' or 'BAM Ireland'.

There may be some discordance in the figures quoted in the text. Much of this story has unfolded in public forums such as Oireachtas committees, the floor of the Dáil or through daily newspapers. On some occasions, people may have misspoken; on others, it wasn't always clear what exactly was covered by the figures they were quoting. Most of these errors were minor and subsequently corrected elsewhere or overtaken by events, but as a result some of the figures in the text may not match up.

Preface

In 2018, I was working as a health journalist when rumours reached me of fresh problems at the national children's hospital.

Conceived years earlier to provide world-leading care for the nation's children, the project aimed to bring three of Dublin's existing hospitals under one roof. It had had a long and controversial history, marked by infighting, political machinations, resignations and money issues – all this before a brick was laid. The location had been changed once, but planning permission to build it southwest of the city centre, at the western end of St James's Hospital, had been granted two years earlier.

Now, as construction was due to get underway, I started hearing the most concerning stories. How the bill for the project was increasing by millions of euro every week. How the final cost of a hospital that started with a €650 million price-tag was now heading for well over €1 billion. How, if this continued, the building could become the most expensive hospital in the world.

While the public remained blithely in the dark, officials in several government departments were aware of the problem, I was told. Some even had a nickname for the increasingly grandiose project – the Edifice Complex.

At the time, I was living nearby. I would often cycle past the site hoardings, gaily decorated with computer-generated images showing happy patients and doctors inside the clean-edged concrete and glass of a brash building. There was a panel illustrating the timeline of the project, which was regularly updated, yet always seemed to be out of date as deadlines constantly slipped.

Four years earlier, I had toured the site, then a jumble of old buildings and overgrown patches of weeds, in the company of the project director. Together, looking over the area from an elevated vantage point, we tried to imagine the giant building that was to arise on this spot. Ireland's biggest construction project, it was thought. A cutting-edge hospital for the sickest children; it was hard not to be excited at this impending symbol of the country's modernisation.

After that visit, the site was cleared and an enormous hole was dug for the foundations of the hospital. But for a long time, and with apologies for the punning, nothing concrete appeared above the hoardings. Something was amiss.

Hearing rumours of the latest overspend, I tried to find out more. To write the story, I needed a figure for the estimated cost of the project. However, no one would provide one. My enquiries were stonewalled, at first by the development board running the project and then by the Department of Health. No firm information was available, I was told.

I kept asking over the months that followed, but was assured there was no cause for concern. All the while, the drumbeat of rumours among my sources grew louder. Finally, in December 2018, the exact figures for the overrun were set down in a cabinet memo, which was leaked to one of my *Irish Times* colleagues in Leinster House. In just six weeks, the officially cited cost of the project had grown by €400 million, the newspaper reported. And further increases were likely.

These were telephone-book numbers, in an era when telephone directories still existed. Their revelation triggered a political firestorm. A plethora of reports and investigations was ordered. The government of the time tottered but ultimately survived. Construction started. And the cost of the hospital continued to go up – a lot faster than the building itself.

Fast forward almost a decade, and the cost is officially estimated at €2.24 billion, though few would be surprised if the final bill reached €3 billion. A project that was promised over 20 years ago is only now approaching an end. The completion date at St James's has been delayed almost 20 times.

I was irked when no one would give me the information I knew existed about the cost overrun back in 2018, and angry when the shocking truth emerged. How maddening that this has been allowed to happen, that ordinary citizens are once again footing the bill for what looks like official ineptitude. How might all that wasted money have been spent? How many more children could have been treated in a hospital that was delivered promptly, instead of a generation late? And if the hospital costs this much to build, how much will it cost to run?

I am also curious *how* this happened. In my career as a journalist, I often came across examples of public waste – shoddy designs, bloated tribunals, pointless pet projects. But nothing on this scale. How is it, I wondered, that we in Ireland so often fail to stay within budget and on deadline on these projects? Is this the reason our infrastructure is lacking, just when it is needed for an expanding population? Can something be learned from the long, unfortunate history of the children's hospital? Or are we doomed to repeat the mistakes made when it was conceived, planned and built?

Nobody set out to deliver an overpriced hospital. Nobody, I believe, deliberately sought to complete the project a generation late. Yet that is what happened. The reasons for this are complex, I found. Hubris, overoptimism, hurry, carelessness and self-interest all played a part.

The story of the national children's hospital, in all its twists and turns, its shocks and reverses, fascinates and appals in equal measure. It is a story about Dublin, and great rivalries in a small place. About promises that were made to a generation of children who, ultimately, were let down by the delays that occurred. It touches on medicine and money, obviously, but also politics, religion, academia and business. Current headlines tell us only part of the story; the project's problems have their roots in decisions and events from years, even decades, ago.

Most of all, this story is about people; families who have been let down too often before, and whose children have had to wait far too long for the world-class hospital in which they were promised they would receive treatment. I hope this book helps to explain why and points a way for the state to do better next time.

Paul Cullen
August 2026

1

'This is wow'

If you want to properly understand the national children's hospital, the place to do this is from a balcony high in the atrium.

It is dizzying up here, perched under an engineered glass dome designed to maximise natural light across the centre of the building, four floors up from the entrance. Below me is the space that will become the beating heart of what is Ireland's largest public building, and its most expensive and controversial.

In time, this vast area will fill with people from all over Ireland: sick children and their families, medical and operations staff, and countless other visitors and volunteers. Regular attenders will hasten down the brightly colour-coded routes to get to clinics and rooms on other floors; new arrivals will make their first port of call the large reception desk offset to the left of the entrance. Every day, the air will fill with the sound of over a thousand voices reflecting the breadth of the hospital experience: young and old, upbeat and fearful, jocular and serious.

On the day of my visit in May 2026, though, this space is eerily silent save for the sound of beeping alarms. The only people traversing the tiled ground-floor concourse are building workers and delivery staff kitted out in hard hats, high-vis jackets and plastic shoe-covers. The planned shops and food outlets along the concourse are boarded up and empty. While the building looks complete to my untrained eye, the hospital isn't open yet, isn't even finished yet, and an opening date has not been set.

The emptiness makes it easier to comprehend its main structural elements. The concourse far below me forms the spine of the hospital, running the length of it, almost as long as Dublin's Grafton Street. The 'hot block' off it is where the main action of a hospital takes place on the lower floors – the emergency department, operating theatres, laboratories and so on. Above this area, on the three uppermost floors, is the oval-shaped ward block, where up to 380 sick children will be accommodated in single rooms, all with exterior views. Running off to the sides of the building are a series of 'fingers', colour-coded again, accommodating day rooms, therapy spaces and mental-health services. A double-storey car park lies hidden underneath the hospital, along with the maintenance and plant facilities.

The real meaning of the building can be gleaned not from these constituent parts of concrete, glass and steel but from the fresh air in front of me – four storeys of it rising up from the entrance area and three more above me. This is dead space that would never exist in a private facility. The enormous, impressive atrium of the National Children's Hospital is the clearest expression that this is a statement building, designed to boost the morale of the citizens. It is also the plainest indication of why this hospital has cost so much money and taken so long to build.

'This is the sort of thing you see in Dubai,' my guide for the day remarks. 'You can't treat patients there or teach staff. It is essentially wasted space.'

There are other hints of this no-expense-spared attitude – the 'biome' above my head, a three-storey metal and glass 'diagrid' structure encapsulating the lifts and stairs; the extensive use of granite cladding on the exterior; the multi-curved silver aluminium roof installed by German engineers; generous play areas between each finger of the building; automatic guided vehicles tasked with delivering medicines and food throughout the hospital; the 'meadow garden' at the end of the concourse; the state-of-the-art hydrotherapy pool and gyms installed on level three.

'This is wow. I beg anyone to contradict me,' my guide says. 'Obviously, a hospital is a place that can be distressing for many. But you can see how this design is trying to take the edge off that.'

I thought back to remarks made by Lucy Nugent, chief executive of Children's Health Ireland, a few months earlier. 'Imagine a world where stepping into a children's hospital feels less like entering a place of illness and more like walking into a space designed for wonder, healing, hope and possibility, where play is woven into every corner,' she told the Oireachtas health committee.

'Imagine a world where robots glide quietly down hallways delivering meals and supplies and there is digital clinical monitoring freeing nurses to spend more time at a child's bedside, where interactive walls turn waiting areas into adventures and gardens and sensory spaces help calm anxious minds.

'In this new hospital, technology and compassion work hand in hand. Families stay close in thoughtfully designed spaces, treatments can happen faster and more gently and even the hardest days are softened by surroundings built with children in mind.

'It is not just a new hospital; it is a transformation in how care feels, where imagination becomes part of the medicine.'

I found Nugent's vision for the hospital compelling. Surely this is what happens when you marry twenty-first-century health technology with a colossal budget? When Europe's fastest-growing economy for much of this century sets its mind to improving the lot of its children? When the very best staff get to pool their expertise under one roof?

But then I thought about how long it had taken to get here and I wasn't so certain. My oldest child is the same age, give or take a few weeks, as the Health Service Executive (HSE), set up in 2005 to transform the running of the health service. My second was born weeks before the decision was first made to build a single national children's hospital, two decades ago.

Both are adults now, and will never be treated here. I'm happy that they hardly ever required the services of any hospital when they were growing up. But I would have been happier if this hospital had been there for them should an emergency have arisen.

And what of sick children, and those with complex needs, who required the best of services, for whom this hospital was promised? And their discovery that it wouldn't arrive for years? I have met a number of them over the past six months, while I was researching this book. Clara (not her real name), for example, told me how, when she was growing up, she constantly dreamed of the shining new hospital in which her treatment would be delivered.

Diagnosed with cystic fibrosis at six months, she gained an early familiarity with care facilities. Much of her childhood was spent being ferried in and out of Our Lady's Hospital for Sick Children in Crumlin where, she says, staff delivered 'unbelievable care' in very trying conditions.

At first, all she required was an annual assessment but by the age of 11, her condition had worsened and she needed inpatient treatment. 'It was the scariest place I had ever been, even with my dad bedded down on the ground beside me. It was so loud, and there was no privacy.'

She remembers how her room had windows both to the ward and to the next room. 'You'd be resting quietly and suddenly some five-year-old would be staring at you through the window.' The bathroom was shared with other patients, many of them highly contagious. Clara, whose condition made her extremely vulnerable to infection, picked up a series of superbugs in hospital. Her condition continued to worsen.

Back then, at the start of this century, her father, along with other parents of children attending Crumlin, began campaigning for a new children's hospital. More importantly for her, when she turned 11 in 2012, Crumlin built new suites for vulnerable children. 'They were beautiful, bright rooms and I thought, *This is good*. And then I found out there were only four. You had to be really lucky or really sick to get one.'

The hospital was trying to fit as much as it could into an old building, while at the same time trying to meet ever-rising demand. Clara remembers how a child's cot was put into one room because the door didn't open enough to allow for a proper bed.

She got sicker as she grew older, spending up to nine weeks at a time in hospital, but the suites weren't always available. She remembers spending time in 'a little cage' with a tiny window, six feet off the ground, and having to use a commode in the room rather than running the risk of using a shared bathroom.

The promised new hospital failed to arrive in time for Clara. 'As a small child, I thought I would eventually be treated in the new children's hospital,' she tells me. 'But at 13, I realised I was never going to see it.'

Despite the setbacks, her story has a happy ending. At 18, she moved over to adult services and was treated in the modern new cystic fibrosis centre built at St Vincent's Hospital. Better still, she got on a clinical trial for new drugs to treat her condition that transformed her life.

'They have made an unbelievable difference. I was very sick, not able to walk, needing oxygen, being in hospital for nine months in the year. Now, it is like night and day – I can do almost everything. And as new drugs are developed, there are fewer side-effects.'

Inspired by the impact on her life of these new treatments that target the genetic defect that causes cystic fibrosis, she decided to study genetics in college. Having recently completed her degree, she plans to undertake further study.

The new children's hospital was planned for children like Clara, but because of the delay in building it, she and many others have aged out. Now 25, Clara finds it incredible that the building has taken so long to complete.

'It won't be for me, now,' she tells me. 'But I really hope it becomes a place where a new generation of children feel they can get better, where the rooms are clean and they can enjoy privacy. Being in hospital, after all, is the most uncomfortable time of your life.'

We had reached the upper floors of the atrium by taking one of the sleek glass-walled lifts at the entrance. Now our tour continues downwards on foot. Trekking down miles of aisles, we visit patient bedrooms, operating theatres, play spaces and outdoor gardens. It doesn't take long to put down the day's 10,000 steps. A Luas tram flashes by a window, showing how well served the hospital is by public transport.

I am reminded of a department store, moments before the January sales rush is due to start. The lights are on everywhere, the wall clocks tell the right time and all surfaces are as clean as a whistle. The plants and trees are just so; someone has to ask if they are real (they are). Yet, I thought, this space wasn't due to open for months, maybe even a year.

At the time of my visit, some individual floors have been handed over to the body responsible for delivering the hospital, the National Paediatric Hospital Development Board (NPHDB), which is readying them for patients. Other floors remain the responsibility of the building contractor, BAM, because the development board says they are not ready to be accepted. This is the latest instalment of a row that has been going on for almost a decade, wherein the blame for soaring costs and ever-lengthening delays is shuttled back and forth between the contractor and its client.

On our visit, we pass various flashpoints of the dispute –

allegedly squeaky doors, a ventilation system that was considered too noisy, square vents in operating theatres that were replaced with circular ones, the reworking of cabling behind ceiling panels, emergency sign panels that had to be moved, changes to the lift cabling.

Individually, these issues seem minor, but when multiplied across over 6,000 rooms, 24 lifts or 22 operating theatres, I can see how costly they must be to remedy. Changes invariably have knock-on effects. Adjust the door seal in an operating room and the air pressure needs to be reset. Shift a socket and a whole heap of wiring has to be moved. Reposition the air conditioning and you have a draught. This is a highly 'intelligent' building; a simple fault like a broken light-bulb triggers a warning alert on its computer systems.

Back down at the entrance, we come across a mammoth object tightly covered in a tarpaulin, with a sign on it saying 'client equipment'. Apparently, it's some kind of toy animal that will be suspended in the atrium for the enjoyment of visiting children. The beast is another victim of the row, left waiting in its package until some arrangement is made to hang it in its proper place.

Two months earlier, in March 2026, the head of the project made one of his regular appearances before politicians, providing updates on progress.

David Gunning, chief officer of the development board, had just read through his prepared statement at the health committee, but then he asked to make an addendum to it.

These sessions have taken on a predictable shape over the years. At each meeting, Gunning announces a further delay in completion of the hospital. The politicians present express shock. Gunning blames BAM for failing to resource the project properly. Later in the day, BAM's public relations company releases a statement, rejecting culpability for delays and blaming them instead on design changes demanded by the development board.

Rinse and repeat. This routine has happened again and again. At least on this occasion, there was good news. In his statement, Gunning said that two weeks earlier BAM had committed to substantially completing the project by the end of the following month. The assurance was given at the highest level, to the minister for health in a meeting with the chief executive of BAM's Dutch parent company, Royal BAM. An end to the project was finally in sight.

But then, Gunning read the addendum, updating the committee on a communication received from BAM the previous day. The 30 April 2026 date would not in fact be met. Another substantial completion deadline would be missed. 'This is obviously a huge disappointment,' he acknowledged, 'as BAM has already delayed the substantial completion date 18 times.'

The TDs in the room shook their heads, I suspect more in sorrow than anger. Sinn Féin's David Cullinane described the news as 'a bombshell' but corrected himself immediately: 'It is not a bombshell because nobody believed that it was going to be met in the first instance. Clearly, from the data provided even for this meeting, that was not going to be the case.'

Cullinane has been his party's health spokesman since 2020.

In that time, he has known only delay in relation to the children's hospital. 'The project has been a disaster from start to finish,' he summarised.

Other TDs joined in the expressions of disappointment. Some deplored a lack of information. Questions were asked, figures provided. After a few hours, lunchtime was looming and the meeting drew to a close.

The theatre was over – until the next time. Once again, the development board had blamed its main builder for a delay. Later in the day, BAM issued yet another statement rejecting this accusation. In the crossfire of allegation and counter-allegation, no one else was any the wiser.

Like most people, I struggle to decide where right lies in this row. Touring the near-complete hospital, though, I could see its impact everywhere. A hospital that looks ready is subject to countless snags, the causes of which are disputed. The occupation of separate floors by the development board and BAM reminds me of the US and the Soviet Union during the Cold War, two superpowers at loggerheads over the hospital universe. No doubt their argument will be settled at some stage, perhaps in court or through mediation. Thereafter, it will be forgotten.

As a health journalist with *The Irish Times*, I wrote often about the hospital. More recently, I tracked the history of the project for this book. By any reading, the hospital's problems are older than any row between a builder and its client. Overspending, delays and underestimation of costs occurred well before BAM got involved.

The problems of today were set in train many years ago. And they aren't just about the building of a hospital, but about the way children's health has been provided; about the way hospitals are run. And about how Ireland is run.

One minister I interviewed summarised the problems of this hospital as 'the wrong design, on the wrong site, contracted in the wrong way and built by the wrong main contractor'. The question I wanted to answer was how this came to be.

THE NATIONAL CHILDREN'S HOSPITAL IN NUMBERS

- 12 acres devoted to hospital, equivalent to 6 soccer pitches
- 7 storeys at its highest, comprising approximately 160,000 square metres of accommodation, including the two-storey car park
- 6,150 rooms
- 380 individual inpatient rooms, each with an en suite and bed for a parent/guardian to sleep near their child
- 93 day beds
- 22 operating theatres and procedure rooms
- 1,000 underground car parking spaces (675 of these for families which can be pre-booked)
- 31 emergency spaces outside the emergency department, supported by a concierge
- 1 rooftop helipad
- 4 acres of outdoor areas and gardens
- 14 gardens and internal courtyards – including an elevated 'Rainbow Garden' which is the length of Croke Park
- 1 paediatric outpatient and urgent-care centre at Connolly Hospital in Blanchardstown
- 1 paediatric outpatient and emergency care unit at Tallaght University Hospital
- 52-unit family accommodation unit, Ronald McDonald House, adjacent to the hospital
- Providing treatment for children up to the eve of their sixteenth birthday, with children already in the system treated up to the eve of their eighteenth birthday.
- Almost 60,000 pieces of equipment
- 40 children's health specialties
- Over 5,000 staff

2

An Avoidable Death

'It is the view of the panel that if Róisín's operation had gone ahead as planned, the likelihood of her survival would have been greater.'
Report of the panel reviewing the events surrounding the death of Róisín Ruddle, published by the Department of Health, February 2005

'We have no doubt at all but had Róisín been given the chance for life on the morning of June 30, 2003, she would be still with us.'
Róisín Ruddle's parents, Gerard Ruddle and Helen Quain, responding to the findings of the report

June 2003: two tiny children, two serious and complex health conditions requiring urgent treatment. One bed. Doctors at the intensive-care unit of Our Lady's Hospital for Sick Children in Crumlin faced an impossible choice.

The hospital didn't have enough specialist nurses, so of 21 beds in the unit, only 13 remained open. Even in the part of the unit where the sickest children were treated, there was funding for eight beds but only enough skilled nurses to cover seven of them. Seven urgent heart operations had been cancelled so far that year, because there weren't enough specialist nurses.

While these staff shortages were the result of a worldwide scarcity of intensive-care nurses, they were exacerbated by changes to the way Irish staff were trained. Several years earlier, the training period for a paediatric ICU nurse was increased from four to seven years, leaving a vacuum that the hospital had failed to address.

Crumlin hospital was also short of funding. In preceding weeks, 25 beds had to remain closed so it could stay in budget. Intensive care, where five nurses were needed on the roster each day to staff every bed around the clock, was where the pressures were felt most acutely.

Temple Street Children's Hospital, across the city on Dublin's northside, had free beds in its intensive-care unit. Perhaps a child could be transferred there, thereby creating room in Crumlin. Or perhaps not; these children were very sick, and unlikely to be suitable for ambulance transfer. No contact was made.

So a grim choice was required between the two sick infants, both of whom were admitted around the same time. One would be treated, the other sent home to await a new date for surgery.

Bubbly two-year-old Róisín Ruddle had arrived up from Kilfinny in County Limerick the day before with her parents, Gerard and Helen. Because she was scheduled to undergo heart surgery, she required the care of two intensive-care nurses.

In her short life, Róisín had grown well used to waiting. Born with a complex congenital heart defect, she was just a few hours old when it was discovered that she needed urgent surgical intervention. Five days passed before a slot could be found for the first emergency operation on her heart, then just the size of a strawberry.

'These first five days turned out to be a "crash course" on what it is to be the parents of a "heart baby" and with it the realisation that from here on our child would be in the care and expertise of the medical profession,' her parents would recall much later, after they had become a national news story.

That operation was a success. For 18 months, she was like all little girls of her age, 'taking part in the hurly-burly of a young life', according to her parents. Then the difficulties caused by her condition became evident and, with them, the need for further medical intervention.

As she grew out of babyhood, Róisín's condition deteriorated – her complexion turned blue, she became short of breath, unsteady on her feet. In March 2003, doctors decided she needed a Glenn shunt, a form of heart surgery for babies born with an issue that doesn't allow normal blood flow through their heart. The procedure redirects blood flow from the upper body directly to the lungs, bypassing the right side of the heart. It gives their one fully functioning ventricle relief and helps them get more oxygen into their blood.

Though a further operation was deemed necessary, this would 'carry her 20 to 30 years without further intervention, and even then the prognosis for her is very good', her parents were given to understand. Medical staff were encouraging; the couple recalled one telling them: 'She might not be a footballer, but she may well be a computer expert.'

Weeks passed but no procedure was scheduled. Róisín's anxious parents, watching their child struggle with her condition at home, rang the hospital repeatedly looking for a date. Slots were limited; there were no dedicated paediatric heart surgeons in Ireland. Operations on children were performed by doctors from the Mater adult hospital, visiting Crumlin for a few sessions a week.

Finally, after three months, the surgical team said it was ready to operate. On a Wednesday in late June, Róisín travelled up to Dublin again for pre-operative tests. Notwithstanding her condition, she had to stay strapped in her car-seat for four hours on the way up. The journey home took five hours, after her parents got caught up in a traffic jam caused by a pop concert.

The following Sunday, she again made the arduous trip to Crumlin and was admitted. Surgery was scheduled for the following day. Her drip was inserted. Róisín fasted overnight. Her parents, by her bedside, endured a sleepless night, but they knew it would be worth it once the shunt was installed.

That Monday, the family waited from early morning for the surgical team to arrive. At 11 o'clock her parents were given the bad news; there were no beds available for Róisín because emergencies had come in. The hospital was short the complement of nurses it needed in intensive care. The other child awaiting a bed was admitted. There was no room for Róisín.

At the last minute, her surgery was deferred. Doctors had made the unenviable choice forced on them by the lack of nurses to care for her post-operatively. Róisín was discharged from the hospital that same day, having been deemed well enough to travel home. With her parents, she returned to Kilfinny. 'Four car journeys over a period of five days ... no parallel anywhere', according to her parents.

At home, her parents put Róisín to bed but she woke them shortly after midnight. Within an hour, she developed seizures and became rigid and pale. The GP arrived and tried to resuscitate her but without success. She was pronounced dead at 1.45 a.m. on the Tuesday morning.

Another victim, another health scandal – Ireland's health service had seen many of them. Minister for health Micheál Martin described Róisín's death as a tragic event and ordered an internal inquiry. This produced a chronological account of what happened and drew attention to the shortage of nurses, but did not make recommendations. Later, a second, independent inquiry would be commissioned.

The surgeon due to perform the operation, Freddie Wood, warned that more children would die if the staffing problems in Crumlin were not resolved. People wondered how, at the height of the Celtic Tiger, a child could die within 24 hours of being discharged from hospital.

The number of heart operations postponed increased rather than fell; in 2004, almost half of 40 postponements were due to staff shortages. One of the children affected was gowned and ready for surgery when his operation was deferred. Crumlin remained 33 short of the specialist intensive care nurses it needed.

The independent report was delayed as the team conducting it struggled to find dates when they were free to meet. It was published, 18 months after Róisín's death, in February 2005. There was no medical evidence that the trips she took were detrimental to her health, it found, while adding that frequent long journeys were 'not ideal for patients with heart conditions'. Róisín would have had a greater chance of survival had the surgery gone ahead, according to the report.

Hospital management was squarely blamed for 'insufficient focus' and a lack of urgency in dealing with the problem of nursing shortages. The Department of Health was also aware of the problem, the report noted: 'The shortage of specialised nurses was predictable from the mid-1990s and this does not appear to have been seen by management at the time as a priority issue warranting significant management attention.'

Resolving issues in this highly critical aspect of the hospital's activities was left to the director of nursing, with no active support from senior managers. No one in the hospital had full-time responsibility for recruiting nurses.

Róisín's parents were left with their unimaginable loss, their unanswered questions, their what-ifs. At one point, they were told by the hospital that agency nurses were available, if funding was available. The treatment delays endured by their daughter led them to believe that waiting lists were a factor that contributed to her fate.

'We have no doubt at all but had Róisín been given the chance for life on the morning of June 30, 2003, she would be still with us,' they said in a statement issued in February 2005. But this chance was 'denied her and, as a consequence, a damnation on us, her parents, who put our misplaced trust in the health system'.

3

The Germ of an Idea

'The Republic guarantees religious and civil liberty, equal rights and equal opportunities to all its citizens, and declares its resolve to pursue the happiness and prosperity of the whole nation and of all its parts, cherishing all of the children of the nation equally.'

Proclamation of the Irish Republic, 24 April 1916

'The children's hospitals were the pits, really.'

Gerry Loftus, former professor of paediatrics at the University of Galway

The man behind the idea of a single national children's hospital is in a reflective mood when I interview him in the kitchen of his south Dublin home on a winter morning. Brendan Drumm, former head of the Health Service Executive, is retired now, his and his wife Marion's time largely taken up with the care of grandchildren, gardening and looking after his family homestead in County Leitrim.

Affable and soft-spoken, Drumm possesses the happy knack of being in the right place at the right time. Starting secondary school in 1968, for example, he found himself in the first cohort in Ireland to avail of free education.

That opened the way for him to study medicine in University College Galway. After graduating, he decided to become a paediatrician, for which he needed to train abroad. Twenty-five rejected applications later, his dream looked as if it was fading. Then, one day, out of the blue, a letter arrived from Toronto's Hospital for Sick Children offering him a trainee place.

The offer might have resulted from someone else dropping out at the last moment, he suspects – right place, right time again. 'In any event, it was a life-changing event. I ended up spending eight years at 'Sick Kids', one of the top three children's hospitals in the world,' he tells me over a cup of warming tea.

His spell in Canada would have a huge impact on the development of health services in Ireland, but not for another few decades. At the time, Drumm's training in paediatric gastro-enterology coincided fortuitously with major scientific break-throughs in the specialty.

Nearing the end of the twentieth century, stomach ulcers were the single major cause of severe illness in adults in developed countries. They tended to be chronic and there was no cure. It had long been assumed that ulcers were caused by excess acid in the stomach. Then, in 1984, two Australian doctors suggested they might be caused by bacteria. The idea was met with great scepticism but eventually won the pair a Nobel prize.

'I began thinking that children would be the ideal group in whom to evaluate this hypothesis,' Drumm explains. 'When we investigated, we found that the bacteria was rarely present in the stomachs of children. But, remarkably, when it was, it was associated with inflammation in the stomach and the presence of ulcers.'

This research was the strongest evidence yet implicating the particular bacterium, *Helicobacter pylori*, as a cause of ulcers. Drumm and his team had three studies published in the *New England Journal of Medicine*.

He describes the discovery as 'life-changing'. Following his appearances in one of the world's most distinguished medical journals, he had his pick of career opportunities and research funding. Still, the lure of home proved irresistible. In 1990, the post of professor and head of paediatrics at University College Dublin and Our Lady's Children's Hospital in Crumlin fell vacant. Drumm got the job.

But was he in the right place at the right time? It didn't seem so. 'The infrastructure in Crumlin was far behind what you would expect. It bore no comparison to what was available in children's hospitals internationally. Conditions in Temple Street Hospital were worse. They would have been unacceptable in any other developed country.'

Drumm sought to develop services across the range of children's specialties, but there was little money in the Ireland of the early 1990s, before the advent of the Celtic Tiger, to invest in health. Paediatrics was the Cinderella of health, and children's hospitals were seriously dilapidated. Improvements could be achieved, he was convinced, only if doctors and managers, and different hospitals, worked together. Far too often, he could see, that wasn't happening.

Children's medicine in Ireland had come a long way in the twentieth century, but starting from a very low base. At its beginning, infectious diseases, driven by overcrowding and poor sanitation, were rampant. Deaths among children were 25 per cent higher in Ireland than in England. Parents could not take it for granted that their children would survive to adulthood. Poverty rates in Dublin in particular were notorious; Charles Cameron, Dublin Corporation's chief medical officer for almost 50 years, said his dream was for every family to have a flush toilet and a tap in their homes.

In 1911, one-fifth of all deaths in Ireland were among children under five – more than 2,000 infants died that year from diarrhoeal illnesses, 1,370 from bronchitis and 945 from 'convulsions'. In 1918–19, the Spanish flu outbreak killed more than 4,000 children aged under 15 in Ireland.

The reality seemed to challenge the 1916 Proclamation's reference to 'cherishing all of the children of the nation equally'. This promise would be frequently quoted in later decades, even if the phrasing is merely a literary device denoting all Irish people.

In the early decades of the new Irish state, children remained at risk from a wide range of infectious diseases. Tuberculosis was the leading cause of death in children in the 1930s. The 1940s saw devastating epidemics of polio. In 1941 alone, almost 1,300 children died in Dublin from a severe epidemic of gastroenteritis.

The health of children across the developed world was transformed as the century progressed. Vaccines were developed to counter the threat posed by polio, measles, tuberculosis and other infectious diseases. In Ireland, spending on health increased in the years after the Second World War, and 450 children's beds were provided in hospitals. More effective medicines, better public health education, the elimination of slums and more state intervention in the health of children also drove improvements in outcomes.

Along with new treatment options for patients, the way health was delivered changed hugely. Children's healthcare moved away from charitable institutions to a more formalised, state-supported system. Sanatoriums and child welfare clinics were opened, and health checks were provided in schools.

Reforms often met huge resistance and the provision of children's health became a touchstone for controversy, most notably during the Mother and Child controversy of 1951. This arose after minister for health Dr Noël Browne proposed the introduction of free healthcare for all mothers and children up to the age of 16. His plans were fiercely opposed by the Catholic Church, which viewed them as encroaching on parental rights, and the medical profession, which feared a threat to income from private practice. Ultimately, the scheme was abandoned and Browne resigned.

Free maternity care and child welfare services were eventually introduced in the 1953 Health Act, which included a pared-down version of Browne's original proposals. By not embracing the universal, no-means-test provisions of the Mother and Child Scheme, the act laid the foundations of the two-tier, public and private system that has defined the Irish health service to this very day.

Ireland spent 4 per cent of its gross national product on health in 1961, rising to 5 per cent in 1970 – approximately half that of Sweden. But even this low outlay was wasteful, because the country had too many hospitals. In 1967, there were 169, most of them inadequately staffed and equipped, according to the landmark Fitzgerald report published by government the following year. They included four children's hospitals, all in Dublin – Crumlin, Temple Street, the National Children's Hospital (NCH) on Harcourt Street and St Ultan's Hospital on Charlemont Street. Also in Dublin, 24 hospitals were treating children alongside adults.

The report by a group of doctors chaired by Professor Patrick Fitzgerald proposed a radical centralisation of hospital care, describing the hospital sector as outmoded and 'a hindrance to good medicine', and calling for a 'considerable reduction' in the number of centres providing acute care.

The group took their cue from a developing international consensus. This held that the path to providing better health services lay in merging smaller hospitals to create larger facilities with greater patient throughput, and therefore more specialised care. But in Ireland, which had high unemployment and poor transport infrastructure, local hospitals were popular in their areas. Even small hospitals provided much-needed jobs. The Fitzgerald report's findings were denounced by local authorities and interest groups. Politicians were loath to interfere, fearing the same backlash dished out to the report.

In any case, there was little funding available for building new infrastructure. Almost a decade on from the publication of the report, the state's entire capital expenditure on the building of hospitals amounted to just IE£16 million (€134 million in today's currency and values), some of it provided as loans or donated by the Irish Hospitals' Sweepstake, a lottery that generated funds for the health service from the 1930s to the 1980s.

The unwillingness to countenance change drew a withering verdict from paediatrician Barry O'Donnell in November 1975: 'Ease of access is no substitute for prolonged hospitalisation, residual disability or a dead patient,' *The Irish Times* reported him saying at a public meeting on reform of the hospital sector. Calling for the amalgamation of all children's beds on the southside of Dublin in Crumlin, O'Donnell said the government's criterion seemed to be that hospitals 'should be established within sight of the polling station'.

From the 1980s, international agencies such as UNICEF and the Organisation for Economic Co-operation and Development (OECD) began publishing regular reports comparing health outcomes and systems in different countries. These exposed Ireland as a relative laggard on health among developed countries. In 1982, life expectancy in Ireland was 73 years, according to the OECD. This was three years lower than in Sweden, where children's care was free and universal.

But infant mortality – deaths among children aged under one – had dropped sharply, from 29.3 deaths per 1,000 births in 1960 to 11.1 in 1980. By 1981, there were no deaths from scarlet fever or whooping cough (pertussis) in Ireland, and only two from measles. Less than 3 per cent of deaths, 916 in total, were of children under five.

The rate of improvement in children's health slowed towards the end of the twentieth century. In 1982, Irish child mortality rates were almost 60 per cent higher than Sweden's. Vaccine uptake plateaued; Ireland had the third lowest rate of immunisation against measles in 1999, and the fourth lowest rate of immunisation against diphtheria, tetanus and whooping cough, an OECD report found.

St Ultan's had closed, but conditions in the three remaining children's hospitals were deteriorating as buildings crumbled. Staff did their best, but investment was urgently needed.

All the while, pressure on services was growing. Ireland had the youngest population in western Europe. From a low of 672,000 in 1951, the population of under-15s increased to 1,008,000 in 1981. High emigration and declining fertility rates saw this figure fall back to 780,000 by the year 2000, before it rose again to over 1 million in 2011.

Irish children had less access to specialist treatment than anywhere else in Europe. There were 16,666 children for every paediatrician in Ireland, according to the 1993 *Paediatrics in Europe* report. Only Britain came close, with a ratio of 12,222 children to each paediatrician. In 12 other countries, the ratio was under 3,000 to one.

Children's hospitals came under tremendous pressure as waiting lists grew and emergency patients ended up on trolleys instead of beds. Doctors working in these hospitals knew that changes were needed urgently.

'The children's hospitals were the pits, really,' Gerry Loftus, a former professor of paediatrics at the University of Galway, tells me in an interview. 'Temple Street was a renovated row of old Georgian houses that had been knocked together,' says Loftus, who trained in

Dublin before spending five years working in London. 'The place was a rabbit warren; you went up and down, in and out all day. The individual cubicles for babies were like small horse boxes. There was no thought that parents might ever want to stay with their sick children.

'Crumlin, meanwhile, was these big, long wards, with small cubicles for children, and some open, multi-bedded areas. It was clear that both hospitals were completely unsuitable.'

A move for Temple Street had been on the cards since 1969; the rebuilding of Crumlin was proposed in 1972 and the transfer of the NCH to another hospital site was mooted in 1981. And yet nothing happened for decades to any of these plans, largely because the country was broke for much of this time.

The doctors working in these hospitals became increasingly frustrated and impatient. Thoroughly sick of toiling in dilapidated conditions, wrestling with ever-growing patient lists, they began to speak out.

In the early 1990s, when Brendan Drumm returned to Ireland, almost 60 paediatricians were working in the Irish health service, most of them in and around Dublin. Many of them, like Drumm, had trained overseas and were appalled by the disrepair in Irish hospitals.

Compared to adult medicine, paediatrics was a relatively new specialty. Initially, children's care was sandwiched between adult and maternity medicine, but its perceived value grew during the twentieth century with greater recognition of the achievements of paediatricians in reducing newborn, infant and child mortality rates. In Britain, paediatricians formed their own association in the

1920s, with the Irish Paediatric Association dating from 1933 (in contrast, child protection societies in both countries date from the nineteenth century).

Recognising the shortcomings in children's health, members of the Faculty of Paediatrics of the Royal College of Physicians held a series of meetings to agree a future direction. In 1993, their conclusions were drawn together in a groundbreaking report, *Recommendations for Dublin Paediatric Services*.

Drumm played a central role in organising these meetings, drawing heavily on his experiences in Toronto. The Canadian city had one primary-care hospital for children in the 1980s for a population of almost 4 million people, and still has only one today. With a high throughput of patients, its doctors developed great expertise in specific areas of treatment, and built up huge research programmes and clinical trials.

'As a result, doctors came from all across the world to train and work there,' Drumm explains. 'You even had paediatricians arriving from London, despite the fact that it was a much bigger city.'

In their report, the Irish paediatricians set aside their traditional affiliations and united to call for a merger of the three remaining Dublin children's hospitals – Our Lady's Hospital for Sick Children in Crumlin, Temple Street Children's Hospital and the NCH in Harcourt Street – in order to provide a comprehensive range of specialised services for children in one location.

Expertise in children's medicine needed to be centralised to avail of economies of scale, they said, because the numbers of children with specific conditions was 'nearly always individually rare'. The report cited international studies showing an improved survival rate for children with cancer, severe lung and heart disease, and kidney failure in a single larger unit, rather than where services were split between sites. Dividing the workload between Dublin's three hospitals militated against trainees developing proper surgical expertise.

For all these reasons, the group unanimously recommended the creation of a single large children's hospital providing tertiary services, while two smaller units would provide secondary care.

Tertiary care is not a term that easily reveals its meaning. It refers to centres operating at the highest level, delivering the most complex advanced care for the sickest patients. So, for example, a patient with a heart issue might see a GP in primary care, be referred to a specialist in secondary care and be operated on by a cardiac surgeon in a tertiary hospital.

'The long-term interests of Irish children would be best served by a single tertiary care centre,' the paediatricians said, rather than continuing with the 'politically feasible' option of parcelling out fragmented care units to various hospitals. 'A single tertiary-care centre is the only feasible answer in Ireland for reasons of the needs of children, economy, the development of excellence, organisation and the future development of the various sub-specialties.' Such a children's complex should be linked to an adult hospital, whether at a single location or 'closely affiliated' to one.

Drumm became outspoken in support of a unified children's hospital. The splitting of services between different locations was both costly and ineffective, he argued. From his own practice in

Crumlin, he knew that small babies with complex bowel problems were being operated on without a gastroenterology support group, when this service was available elsewhere. If services at the three children's hospitals were amalgamated, specialist children's surgeons could be employed instead of relying on adult surgeons to occasionally operate on children.

'The evidence was irrefutable from adult hospitals across the world – the number of cases managed was directly correlated to the quality of outcomes for each condition. This was especially true where surgery was required,' he tells me.

'The corollary of this was that patients attending smaller hospitals performing low numbers of specific interventions were at increased risk of adverse outcomes. In my mind, it was unacceptable that in Dublin, specialised services for children were being provided across three centres.'

Drumm earned a reputation as a straight talker, not afraid to upset vested interests. The Dublin children's hospitals were more concerned about their own interests than the provision of quality care for sick children, he told a conference in July 1995, adding, 'It appears as if the individual paediatric and maternity institutions have, above all else, placed their own survival as the issue of most importance on the agenda.'

The paediatricians had spoken with one voice: there should be one single hospital to treat the sickest children and it should be located alongside an adult hospital. Yet despite their pleas and the generally improving financial situation, successive governments ignored the amalgamation proposal. Instead, they pursued plans to upgrade the existing children's hospitals.

'Nothing happened after the report came out,' Gerry Loftus tells me. 'It was a case of the urgent displacing the important. The service was creaking, so developments had to happen, even if on a stuttering basis. No one was prepared to say stop, and do things differently. The result was piecemeal development.'

Even with Temple Street, the oldest and most decrepit of the children's hospital buildings, various proposals to move it to the nearby Mater site were ignored in favour of small-scale renovations. 'In one way the grand plan has inhibited smaller plans which might remedy the problems,' minister for health Michael Noonan told the Dáil in 1995. 'The cost is huge and I cannot indicate when progress will be made.'

Thus, by the end of the twentieth century, it was clear that the lot of Irish children had improved greatly since independence. However, the progress made in reducing child mortality was largely the result of improvements in vaccines and drug treatments globally. The rate at which outcomes were improving had begun to slow, and Ireland continued to lag behind its European neighbours. Investment was low, despite the obvious needs posed by a crumbling infrastructure. While doctors had suggested the way forward, there was little political appetite for reform. Besides, as would soon become apparent, not every impediment to change could be blamed on lethargic politicians or vested interests outside the health service.

4

'Coming apart at the seams'

Disease and malnutrition were rife in the poorly lit Georgian tenements.
Barry Kennerk, in *Temple Street Children's Hospital: An Illustrated History*

'I oppose this amalgamation on religious principles solely. The faith of Catholic children is of more importance in the eyes of the Catholic Church than any other thing in the world.'
Catholic Archbishop of Dublin Edward Byrne, opposing the amalgamation of St Ultan's Hospital and the National Children's Hospital, December 1935

Dublin has a proud history of children's medicine, tarnished by long-running professional, institutional, religious and academic rivalries. One result of this is a series of messy hospital mergers, of which the current creation of a new national children's hospital from three existing institutions is only the latest.

The city was the first in Britain or Ireland to open a children's hospital. This was hardly an accident, given the levels of poverty and overcrowding, and related prevalence of infectious diseases, for much of the nineteenth and twentieth centuries, but it shows the length of the city's medical heritage.

By the start of this century, and despite its modest size, the city was home to three very different institutions treating children, all of which had outgrown the buildings in which they were housed. Small by international standards, they struggled to provide the specialist care required by the sickest children.

The oldest of these institutions was the National Children's Hospital (NCH) – a misleading name since it was also the smallest. The Dublin Institution for the Treatment of Diseases of Children, as it was originally called, dated back to 1822 – just 20 years after the world's first children's hospital was established in Paris and 30 years before Great Ormond Street Hospital would open its doors in London.

The hospital started life at Pitt Street (now Balfe Street, where the Westbury Hotel is located). One of its founders went on to establish Great Ormond Street, with the support of novelist Charles Dickens among others. Over 4,000 child outpatients were treated at Pitt Street during the first two years. In 1888, after amalgamating with an orthopaedic hospital, the NCH moved to 87 and 88 Harcourt Street, its final home.

Liberal and independent in outlook, the board of the hospital tended to be heavy with prominent figures from the Anglo-Irish aristocracy and the medical profession. A strong training link developed with Trinity College, traditionally Dublin's Protestant university.

Catholic interests sought to establish an institution devoted to the medical care of Catholic children as the Church's fortunes improved during the nineteenth century. In 1872, two female philanthropists founded an eight-bed hospital on Upper Buckingham Street, in Dublin's north inner city. Within four years, the Religious Sisters of Charity had taken over its operation.

Dublin had one of the highest rates of child mortality in the world at the time, and the new institution was located in the heart of its most overcrowded slums. 'Disease and malnutrition were rife in the poorly-lit Georgian tenements,' Barry Kennerk wrote in *Temple Street Children's Hospital: An Illustrated History*:

> Rickets – a deformity of the bones – was so commonplace that it hardly attracted notice and in many cases was caused by a meagre diet, often with skimmed milk or buttermilk which was deficient in Vitamin D. Many Dubliners shared single outdoor toilets which were little more than breeding grounds for flies and parasites. In the evenings they piled into crumbling rooms where typhus fever, spread by lice in their clothing, was inescapable. Outside, a charcoal-smelling fog lingered, brought on by coal fires which choked the lungs, and many babies died with no medical attention of any kind. Broken stairwells and faulty railings ensured that many more succumbed to serious injury and death.

When the hospital's lease expired in 1879, the Sisters of Charity bought the former seat of the earls of Bellomont at 15 Temple Street, still in the north inner city, which became the hospital's permanent home. Adjoining buildings were acquired over the following years, and in the 1930s the Irish Hospitals' Sweepstake funded further expansion.

The ghost of another, long-departed Dublin children's hospital haunts this tale. In 1919, Dr Kathleen Lynn, her life partner Madeleine Ffrench-Mullen and other activists founded St Ultan's Hospital for Sick Infants on Charlemont Street, on the southside of the city, just as a major flu pandemic was sweeping across Europe.

Lynn was a curious mix: eccentric yet driven; a socialist, feminist and republican; an Anglo-Irish Protestant and committed Christian to the end of her life. Determined to provide the most up-to-date care for her child patients, she travelled to hospitals across Europe and the US to learn about new paediatric practices. With her largely female staff at St Ultan's, she introduced many innovative approaches to care, including an electric breast pump, Montessori care, goats' milk and outdoor sunshine wards. As historian Mary McAuliffe has written in *The Diaries of Kathleen Lynn*, staff at St Ultan's led research into child tuberculosis in the 1930s, and were instrumental in the introduction of the BCG (Bacillus Calmette-Guérin) inoculation to Ireland.

Lynn's dream for many years was to amalgamate her hospital with the other southside children's hospital on Harcourt Street to create a truly national institution for children. Lands around St Ultan's were purchased and her friend, the architect Michael Scott, drew up plans for a modern new building.

However, the project ran into opposition from the Catholic Church. Both St Ultan's and the NCH were secular institutions, over which the Church had little direct influence.

The merger never came to fruition, but another of Dublin's children's hospitals, Our Lady's Hospital for Sick Children (Crumlin), has its roots in this controversy. Another Catholic children's hospital had been mooted years earlier by Edward Byrne, archbishop of Dublin from 1921 to 1940. Having witnessed widespread poverty in the inner city when he worked as a curate, Byrne vowed to improve the health of children by building a facility devoted to their needs.

His plan languished until the row erupted over the planned merger of St Ultan's and the NCH. In December 1935, Byrne blocked this proposal for a bigger hospital with liberal governance with a blunt statement opposing the amalgamation on 'religious principles only'. The faith of Catholic children was at risk under a Protestant staff, he warned.

Three years later, Dublin Corporation sold a site in Crumlin to the archbishop of Dublin for the planned new Catholic children's hospital. Although Byrne died in 1940, Éamon de Valera backed his idea, notwithstanding the Fianna Fáil leader's friendship with Lynn. The Second World War intervened, so construction didn't get underway until 1950, with the help of funding from the sweepstake.

Meanwhile on Harcourt Street, the NCH's bed numbers remained small, leading to constant uncertainty over its future. There were talks about moving to St James's Hospital – ironically now the site of the new children's hospital – in 1970 as well as negotiations with Crumlin, but neither came to anything.

With thousands of children moving through its wards over the years – I spent a few nights there myself, having tonsils removed –

the NCH became a much-revered Dublin institution. Among its most renowned staff was Dr Bob Collis, who trained in England and the US before returning to Ireland in the 1930s to work in the NCH and the Rotunda maternity hospital. Collis, a writer and former Ireland rugby international, was instrumental in improving services for premature babies. Collis set up the first dedicated cerebral palsy clinic in Dublin – one of his patients was Christy Brown, author of *My Left Foot*. He volunteered with the Red Cross at the Bergen-Belsen concentration camp after its liberation by Allied troops in 1945, and brought orphaned child survivors to Ireland the following year.

After Lynn died in 1955, St Ultan's struggled on for another few decades. It closed in 1984 and its services were moved to the NCH on Harcourt Street.

But that hospital was also nearing its end. In 1981, the Department of Health had pushed for the NCH to join two Dublin adult hospitals, the Meath and Adelaide, in moving to a new campus in Tallaght, on the southwest fringe of the city. The new entity, an amalgam of Catholic and Protestant hospitals, would have a liberal ethos and serve as a teaching hospital for Trinity College.

The move went ahead and Harcourt Street finally closed in 1998. Its buildings were put up for sale with a price tag of £1.7 million. Today, the Georgian frontage of the old hospital masks a large office block on the site.

As for Temple Street, a government-commissioned report had recommended in 1969 that it should be 'closely associated' with the Mater, an adult hospital nearby. This proposal was not acted on and the hospital's management continued to develop services on the existing site.

Temple Street marked its centenary in 1972 with great pomp, Archbishop John Charles McQuaid celebrating a mass attended by the ageing president Éamon de Valera. Over the following 20 years, the hospital became 'less of a house and more a modern hospital', Barry Kennerk wrote. Its name changed several times, but always contained a reference to Temple Street. It developed training links to both University College Dublin (UCD) and Trinity College Dublin.

In 1984, the Department of Health announced a plan to construct a new hospital to replace the existing buildings on Temple Street. Nothing happened owing to health-service cutbacks. Four years later, the plan was to replace it with a standalone paediatric hospital adjoining the Mater. Again, nothing happened, and whatever investment that had become available was used to upgrade and expand the existing hospital.

The old hospital suffered greatly as the cutbacks continued. 'Temple Street is coming apart at the seams,' a letter-writer to *The Irish Times* complained in October 1988. 'Last year, part of the outpatients department collapsed. Clinics are held in timber huts with leaking roofs and broken windows.'

By the end of the century, the hospital had built on most of its open space. 'Wards and offices tower over the A&E laneway like a ziggurat,' according to Kennerk, and further construction was increasingly confined. 'With little exaggeration,' he wrote, 'there may be a Kango hammer in use on one side of a wall while a scalpel is deployed on the other.'

~

Dr Noël Browne, minister for health from 1948 to 1951, had sought to make the planned Catholic hospital in Crumlin 'subject to proper public or democratic control', according to his memoir, but found that an 'irrevocable agreement' had been made in the 1930s between Archbishop Byrne and the then minister for health, ensuring the hospital would be run by the Church. As a result, the two largest children's hospitals in Dublin, Crumlin and Temple Street, were run with a strongly Catholic ethos.

Opened by Archbishop McQuaid in July 1956, the 300-bed hospital in Crumlin was run by the Daughters of Charity of St Vincent de Paul. 'We called them the French Sisters of Charity,' Gertie McCormack, one of the first non-religious nurses recruited for the new hospital, recalled decades later in an *Irish Times* interview. 'They had the big butterfly hats and we were terrified of them.'

Crumlin expanded considerably in the 1960s and developed training links with University College Dublin, which had deep Catholic roots. The site became increasingly cluttered with each successive extension. 'In all my time there, we never seemed to have enough money or staff,' Professor Maurice Neligan, who carried out heart surgery in the hospital for over 30 years, recalled in an *Irish Times* column in 2009.

Crumlin was 'constantly falling apart,' a senior civil servant tells me in an interview. 'We were bolting things onto part of the hospital that should have been demolished earlier.'

'Despite the affluence of recent years, problems of access and funding still blight the capabilities of the hospital,' Neligan wrote. 'There were times when the cracks could not be papered over and when staff and beds were in such short supply that postponement of treatments and cancellations of operations became inevitable.'

By the start of this century, Crumlin and Temple Street were dilapidated, starved of state funding and heavily reliant on charitable fundraising to survive. Paediatric services in Tallaght were new but enjoyed little clout. The three hospitals were divided by geography, clinical rivalries, academic linkages and religious affiliations. Some consolidation had occurred but more was needed. Staff wanted change, but there was little agreement on where amalgamated services should be provided. The voice of patients – children and their parents – had yet to be heard.

5

'This is not acceptable'

'The defects and deficiencies in the hospital are very great indeed.'

Report by UK health planning expert Dr Ronald Pollock on Crumlin hospital, published December 2002

'We were told not to publish the report or there would be "daggers at dawn".'

New Crumlin Hospital Group parent Louis Roden on the hospital board's attitude to the Pollock report

Linda Dillon moved into the children's hospital in Crumlin the day her daughter was diagnosed with cancer. And ended up staying there for three months.

In 2001, Alice had just turned three. An initial diagnosis of anaemia had turned into something far more serious: neuroblastoma, a rare cancer of the nerve tissue that affects one child in 7,000.

'The doctor said she was going to need a year of chemo, surgery, the divil and all,' Dillon recalls. 'We asked should we take her home, if it was going to be that bad, and he said that wasn't even possible in her condition.'

Dillon is understated, even matter of fact, when we meet in the large reception room of a Dublin hotel. Amid the clatter of cutlery and plates, she describes how the serious illness of a child turned her family life upside down and made a campaigner out of a stay-at-home mother.

While she moved in with her daughter in hospital, her husband Patrick had to give up work to care for their two other children, then aged nine and twelve. That first night, she was put up on a mattress on the floor of the fully occupied cystic fibrosis ward.

'I got my first impression of what the place was like the following morning, when they were wheeling Alice along in a trolley. I thought, *Oh my God, this is so bad. They have the cancer patients hidden away. They are so far down the back of the hospital that they have a line of broken beds along the corridor*.'

A daily routine developed for Linda as Alice underwent her treatment. 'There was this miserable playroom at the end of her ward where the folding beds were stored. Every night, after searching for clean sheets, I and the other parents would roll the beds and mattresses to our children's rooms on the cancer ward, sleep there, and roll them back the following morning. There were two patients to each room, so you might have another mam or dad sleeping on the other side of the floor with their child. You never complained – where was that going to get you?'

Doctors had found a large tumour in Alice's kidney and the cancer had spread to her bone marrow and liver. Initially, her parents were told to expect the worst but the outlook improved as medical staff developed a treatment plan. Thanks to their efforts, she began to thrive.

The room where Alice stayed after her surgery was so small, some of the machines monitoring her progress had to be kept outside the door. 'That was the beginning of me saying this is not acceptable,' Linda says. 'I remember looking out the window at the Dublin mountains and starting to realise that there was this whole other world there. That most people, thankfully, didn't know about this. That it was absolutely insane – how could the hospital be the way it was and no one knew anything about it?

'I said to myself that no matter what happened, whether we left there with or without Alice, there was no way I could walk away from that hospital without doing something. I didn't know then what it would be. I was a mum at home, I wasn't normally a doer, but I felt compelled to do something.'

One wintry Saturday morning in 2002, Linda Dillon and about 30 other parents of children attending Crumlin trooped into an auditorium for a meeting called by consultants at the hospital.

Over the preceding years, children's medicine had been in the news for all the wrong reasons. From 1999, it emerged that Crumlin had stored children's organs after their death, without their parents' knowledge. Amid uproar, it had to apologise to the families of almost 100 children whose organs were kept long after the postmortem examinations on their remains. One child's heart and lungs remained on a shelf in the hospital, five years after the child's death. Up to the mid-1980s, it also emerged, glands had been harvested from thousands of dead children and given to a pharmaceutical company for research.

The organ-retention scandal was to drag on for years. An inquiry would be established in 2000 but was wound up after five years due to lack of progress. Further reports and audits were then commissioned.

Unwelcome though it was, the controversy shone a light on the problems of overcrowding and dilapidation in the hospital, along with its heavy reliance on fundraising. Across children's medicine, new facilities had been promised for years, even decades. In 2001, the government committed to a review of paediatric services nationally, but this was not done until four years later.

Now Brendan Drumm and other doctors, appalled at the deteriorating state of the hospital, resolved to alter that narrative. And they were going to rely on the parents of sick children, carefully handpicked to attend the meeting, to front the campaign for change.

'The doctors told us they couldn't get movement from government so it was now down to us parents to make progress,' Louis Roden, the father of two cystic fibrosis patients at the hospital, recalls.

The parents who attended the meeting set up the New Crumlin Hospital Group, dedicated to the aim of getting the hospital rebuilt. A committee was formed to coordinate the campaign. 'All of us total strangers, all parents of very sick children,' Linda Dillon recalls. 'We called ourselves the 12 apostles.'

'Brendan [Drumm] had been lobbying for better facilities but wasn't making progress. We all agreed the situation was beyond ridiculous that we had to do this,' another parent, Karl Anderson, who was chosen by the parents to chair the committee, tells me.

Anderson, who would go on to work as an advisor to Drumm in the Health Service Executive, was a communications consultant, but most of the parents had no experience in lobbying. 'The thing about parents and lobbying for facilities – there is a very unusual dynamic to it. When your child is sick, you want to get the best care that you can, you want to get treatment, and you want to get the hell out of there,' he explains. 'You want to disconnect from the hospital if at all possible once you're done. Naturally, for some this is not possible as their child may require ongoing treatment during their whole childhood.

'And if your child is *very* sick, say they have a heart condition or ongoing cancer, you don't have the bandwidth to complain. Simply coping takes all your physical and mental energy.'

Parents are often desperately thankful for the efforts of the staff treating their children, he says. 'The last thing you want to do is criticise, for fear that the care that you're going to get will be somehow impacted. As a result, you didn't see the parents of sick children lobbying very often.'

The Crumlin initiative was designed to reverse this tradition of patient quiescence. The parents knew they were in for a long campaign. 'It was never going to be about *our* children. All we could hope was that, perhaps, our grandchildren might benefit if we were successful,' Dillon says.

The parents tried to enlist the support of hospital management. 'I could understand why there hadn't been any change,' Dillon says. 'It was obvious in the way they were talking. They were fluffing around the house, going through the motions. They felt they had to entertain us.'

They looked outside Ireland for help. Funded by a donor whose identity remains secret to this day, the group commissioned a report from a UK expert on health service planning, Dr Ronnie Pollock.

Published in December 2002, Pollock's report delivered a damning account of conditions in the state's largest children's hospital. The buildings in Crumlin were seriously outdated and needed to be replaced, it found. 'The defects and deficiencies in the hospital are very great indeed, and this after heroic efforts over the years to expand and improve facilities,' Dr Pollock told journalists at a press conference to launch the report.

He was scathing about the condition of the hospital. Its intensive-care provision was 'very limited', wards were designed in such a way that they wasted nurses' time, the outpatients department had 'grossly insufficient space' and many of its diagnostic facilities were not 'up to current acceptable standards'.

'I can see hardly any scope for improvement through "patching" the present framework, and absolutely no way in which currently accepted standards can be provided,' he concluded.

The case for new facilities was clear. As Pollock pointed out, attendances by children at the hospital had grown six-fold in 40 years. And in contrast to the 1950s, when children often had to endure long hospital stays on their own, the parents of very sick children now tended to stay with them. Despite this, the report noted, Crumlin had 'virtually no facilities' for parents and relatives, 'either in the form of rest rooms and refreshment facilities or in the provision for overnight stay beside an ill child'.

Linda Dillon, in follow-up media interviews, described the shabby 'rabbit warren of huts and Portakabins' where Alice and other children with cancer were being treated. 'It seemed impossible to think that this was our national children's hospital, the last hope for seriously ill children from all over Ireland,' she tells me.

Crumlin had briefly looked at moving to St James's Hospital nearby, and to Tallaght Hospital, according to an informed source, but nothing came of either idea. For now, redevelopment of the hospital on its existing site seemed to be the preferred option of parents and staff.

While, officially, the chairman of Crumlin hospital was the Catholic archbishop of Dublin, some incumbents tended to take a back-seat role, leaving the running of the facility to a deputy. At this stage, the vice-chairperson of the hospital board was former Dublin city manager Frank Feely.

Avuncular and gregarious, the bushy-browed Feely was once described in a newspaper article as 'bestriding the city like a colossus'. He tended to bestride Crumlin too, taking it upon himself to read his chief executive's reports at board meetings and, as one source put it, sucked 'all the air out of the room'.

He was unenthused by the parents' bid for the limelight. 'His attitude was: "We could maybe get a few curtains for some of the wards. We could paint some of them." This in a situation where parents were sleeping on the floor beside their kids in an open ward,' Anderson recalls.

'This was the level of his acceptance of the problem. It was like we should be grateful for the care our children were getting and should not be complaining. He didn't want any spotlight on conditions in case it affected the hospital's fundraising.'

The parents' group presented its report to the board of the hospital. 'The archbishop didn't turn up,' Roden recalls. 'The rest of them were astounded. Who was this bunch of do-gooders, they wanted to know. We were told not to publish the report or there would be "daggers at dawn". But we published it anyway – left, right and centre.'

Anderson also recalls Feely warning of 'daggers at dawn' if the report was published but adds that nothing came of the threat. 'It spoke volumes for their appreciation of the conditions that parents and their kids were putting up with.'

The parents continued to press their case despite opposition from within Crumlin. Effectively bypassing the hospital board, they appealed directly to politicians. Minister for health Micheál Martin had publicly acknowledged that the infrastructure at Crumlin was unacceptable but the parents wanted action.

'On foot of the report, we got a meeting with Martin,' Anderson says. 'There must have been 20 of his officials at the meeting in his Dáil office. He was very sympathetic and recognised something needed to be done, but offered no deadlines.'

When Diarmuid Martin was appointed archbishop of Dublin in 2004, he made it his business to get involved in the running of Crumlin. Martin, who was to remain archbishop until his retirement in 2020, felt the hospital wasn't functioning properly.

There were, he tells me on a call from Rome, strains between different departments, and between the hospital and its fundraising arm. 'At the board, some members said nothing, while others, who were merely "in attendance", dominated meetings.

'There was a lack of competence. People were on boards for years. In those days, you were made chair if you couldn't get an honorary degree. A man would be there forever if his wife thought it was a good idea for him to get out of the house for a few hours.'

Martin believed he had a legal obligation to act as chairman of the board, even if this upset Feely. Revamping hospital governance would take time, he realised. In the interim, he tried to figure out a future for the hospital, amid differing opinions internally about how it should be redeveloped.

'Mary Harney [who had succeeded Micheál Martin as minister for health] and I did a walk-around in 2004. At that stage, people wanted to stay put. But the building was in poor condition in places. There was nothing we could do. You couldn't run a hospital in a building site.'

Older doctors in the hospital tended to favour a continuation of Crumlin in some form, he says, while younger colleagues were more open to a move. Tensions with Temple Street were evident: 'There wasn't much contact between the hospitals. You had a north–south divide, a feeling that "we're better than you are".'

Meanwhile, the funding relationship between the hospital, a voluntary hospital with its own board, and the HSE and the Department of Health was 'complicated'. 'If you can explain it,' he tells me, 'you can explain the Blessed Trinity.'

Archbishops know a thing or two about hierarchies, but it is the medical pecking order that Martin raises during our conversation, prefacing his remarks with an anecdote about the time he spent in hospital as a child in the 1950s.

He was a patient for three weeks in the old Richmond adult hospital after breaking his leg. 'Four surgeons were caring for my leg and each time they entered the ward, a gong was rung four times. One gong for each of them.'

Traces of the same type of medical hierarchy were evident in Crumlin hospital when Martin began chairing the institution, he says.

Across the city, Temple Street Children's Hospital was older and in even worse condition than Crumlin, but at least it seemed to have a clear plan for the future.

In 2001, in spite of the earlier recommendation by paediatricians for a single tertiary hospital for children, plans were announced for a £268 million (€340 million) development to move Temple Street to the grounds of the Mater adult hospital nearby and to upgrade some of the Mater buildings. With both hospitals set to benefit from the investment, the plan enjoyed overwhelming support among staff and patients.

Professor Michael O'Keeffe, an ophthalmologist at both Temple Street and the Mater and the brother of a Fianna Fáil TD, was a leading advocate for the two hospitals to be united on the one campus. However, the Mater's most prominent supporter was Fianna Fáil's leader, Bertie Ahern, the taoiseach since 1997 and a former employee of the hospital.

Half a century on from when he worked there, Bertie Ahern still has fond memories of the Mater. 'The nuns were decent people, they never caused any problems,' he recalls, ordering a second round of toast to go with his pot of tea.

I'm interviewing the former taoiseach on his home turf, in a hotel in Drumcondra, on a stormy day in December 2025. An extreme weather warning hasn't deterred him from turning up to meet me and, afterwards, attend the local old folks' Christmas party in a reception room of the hotel. Throughout our interview, a succession of retirees, mostly women, come up to shake his hand and wish him well.

After a first job with the Dublin District Milk Board, Ahern served in the accounts department of the Mater from the early 1970s. He worked as assistant accountant of both the public and private hospitals; others have pointed out that he does not have a chartered accountant qualification and have described his role there as more akin to an accounts clerk.

At the private hospital, he tells me, he did 'all the figures', out of which he was offered the role of chief executive. 'But I was a gobshite, you know, I stayed in politics.' Even today, he remembers the sums of money involved in precise terms – 'I was offered 20 grand to be CEO, when a TD was being paid 6,901 pounds.'

He continued to work in the public hospital after he was elected a TD in the 1977 general election. Without his post in the Mater, he might have been forced out of public life by the financial strain involved, he explained in his autobiography, published in 2009. The arrangement with the hospital ended only when he was appointed a minister in 1982.

Ahern recalls the Department of Health commissioning an English consultancy firm in the mid-1970s to model a new hospital at the Mater. 'As part of that, Temple Street, which was falling down, was to become part of the Mater. Limited money was being put into Temple Street. The guys there got very upset when Tallaght was built and Harcourt Street went out there.

'The consultants were worrying about their own positions. Michael [O'Keeffe] was a lovely man but fierce political – Jaysus, he drove me mad. All he wanted was Temple Street on the Mater complex. He didn't like the consultants in Crumlin and they didn't like him. The rows started with the concept of two children's hospitals, one northside and one southside.'

Ahern wanted to see the Mater redeveloped, he tells me, and was 'happy' for Temple Street to be moved there as part of the plan. But he didn't think having one children's hospital was a good idea. One of his daughters was living in Malahide in north Dublin, so if Tallaght was chosen as the site of a single hospital, she would have to bring a sick child all the way to the other end of the county.

Promises had been made about the children's hospitals before, many times. But with Ireland's Celtic Tiger economy in full flow, optimism was growing around the Mater and Temple Street that, this time, the planned new facilities would become a reality.

Construction at the Mater was slated to begin in 2002 and be completed by 2008. Treatment of adults and children would be provided separately but 'back to back' on the new campus, with the two hospitals having separate entrances, according to the Sisters of Charity, who ran Temple Street, and the Sisters of Mercy, who ran the Mater Hospital.

The new children's hospital was to have 170 beds, 38 more than Temple Street at the time. This was well below the 300-bed minimum size for a hospital recommended by the Fitzgerald report in the late 1960s. It also went against the call by paediatricians in 1993 for a single – and necessarily larger – hospital for very sick children.

An application for planning permission was submitted promptly in February 2002. It seemed nothing could stand in the way of the long-awaited and much-needed redevelopment of Temple Street. Government still had to give the final go-ahead, but this wasn't seen as a big obstacle. After all, both Temple Street and the Mater were in Ahern's constituency in the north inner city; the Fianna Fáil leader's dedication to supporting projects in his home patch was unrivalled.

There was only one problem. Campaigning by parents in Crumlin about its shortcomings had pushed the renovation of that hospital up the political agenda. Róisín Ruddle's death had laid bare the deleterious impacts of mismanagement and under-resourcing at the hospital. Micheál Martin, Ahern's party colleague and minister for health, was making positive noises about renovating Crumlin.

It seemed the government was assenting to the redevelopment of two children's hospitals in Dublin at a time of constrained health funding, while the country's paediatricians believed there should be only one. Something would have to give.

6

'It was like Celtic versus Rangers'

'Hospitals are very expensive to build and equip and they could absorb every last euro available.'
Minister for health Mary Harney addressing the Progressive Democrats annual conference, April 2005

'If the decision to call off the new Temple Street is not reversed, it will be a major lost opportunity for children.'
Letter from 22 Temple Street consultants to *The Irish Times* in January 2006, prompted by the HSE's decision to pause plans to move the hospital to the Mater Hospital nearby

'It is difficult for outsiders to understand the level of antipathy that existed between the children's hospitals in Dublin,' retired paediatrician Gerry Loftus remarks in our conversation.

Based in Galway for most of his career, Loftus had a ringside seat for the rivalries that marred children's medicine in the capital. 'You got a lot of institutional chauvinism and hubris, people saying "we're much better than them" or "we've always been hard done by". Proposals were seen through the prism of "my team". It was like Celtic versus Rangers; they've both got a passion, but ... There was such parochialism. It was always a zero-sum game; if one hospital benefited, the other felt it was losing.'

Crumlin and Temple Street, the two largest children's hospitals, were now vying for government support for their redevelopment plans. Relations between them remained glacial. And just as the parents in Crumlin were starting to mobilise, this simmering rivalry hit the headlines.

When the one paediatric urologist in the state retired, it was assumed his post would be filled within a year. But due to rows over the structuring of the post between the three children's hospitals, it had lain vacant. Rather than confront the vested interests, the Department of Health opted to send children needing complex urology surgery to the UK. The row resulted in a much-needed consultant post remaining vacant for seven years, *The Irish Times* reported in March 2003.

The dispute showed that the problems around children's care weren't just about funding, or bricks and mortar. Chronic infighting over resources between the children's hospitals underscored the need for a national review of services, which had been promised some years earlier. Previous moves to centralise haematology and oncology services had also provoked lengthy disputes, although this process was eventually concluded when four children's cancer treatment centres in Crumlin, Tallaght, Galway and Cork were consolidated in Crumlin.

Many sick children have complex conditions that require input from a variety of specialties, so treatment can be problematic when these are provided in different hospitals. Surgery on newborns was split between Temple Street and Crumlin, even for conditions where only a handful of patients were seen every year. A 1998 report calling for all children's surgery to be carried out at one site was ignored.

'The three children's hospitals were always competing for whatever resources were available,' Loftus says. 'Services were split up. If you had a cardiac problem, you had to go to Crumlin, but neurology was split between Crumlin and Temple Street. You had to choose based on service availability, and hope that the specialist service you opted for was the correct choice. The offer was clearly below what it should have been.'

One paediatric surgeon had to work across Tallaght, Crumlin and Temple Street because each of them insisted he attend for at least three sessions a week. 'Anything else would be less than parity of esteem as far as the hospitals were concerned,' a civil servant who tried to mediate that dispute tells me.

To complicate matters further, paediatric cardiac surgery was performed by two surgeons based in the Mater with part-time commitments to Crumlin. 'I'm not sure that best served either adult or child patients,' the civil servant says.

Relations between the different hospitals were often fraught, according to one doctor-turned-administrator who makes the general point that 'medical politics is often more vicious than national politics'.

The Crumlin–Temple Street relationship in particular involved an 'unending institutional dogfight', a Temple Street paediatrician,

Professor Tom Matthews, noted in a candid letter to *The Irish Times* around this time.

Remarking on the many advances he had seen in children's medicine over the preceding decades, Matthews said that 'almost the only blot on an otherwise immensely satisfying medical career was the continuous internecine trench warfare between the children's hospitals'. This was a 'constant background factor, with each side lining up support among the Department of Health, local politicians, ex-patients, parents, etc., making it impossible to remain neutral while working in either children's hospital'.

'I think it was down to jealousy,' says a doctor who worked in Crumlin for many years. 'Crumlin was built only in the 1950s, but it became the biggest hospital, with more national specialties, including cardiac care and cancer. Temple Street was developing its intensive-care unit but had nothing of national status among its sub-specialties.

'As a result of all the sparring, the greatest impediment to advancing paediatrics in Dublin were the paediatricians, not government policy. No one wanted to invest in paediatrics because of this rivalry. My colleagues were cutting off their nose to spite their face.'

As Róisín Ruddle's case showed, dysfunction in children's health could have dire consequences.

'Her case opened up a thing in our minds,' says Linda Dillon. 'Here was an issue: you had children who couldn't be dealt with in one hospital, but there was another hospital, across the city ... Where was the working together in all of this?'

In 2003, Crumlin had just three toilets for 25 children in the oncology ward, where immuno-suppressed patients were in danger of picking up infections. Children were being ferried by taxi to Beaumont Hospital on Dublin's northside for MRI scans. In the years after Róisín's death, staff shortages continued to force the postponement of dozens of heart surgeries planned for very sick children.

Brendan Drumm made a submission to the panel investigating Róisín's death in which he called for the appointment of full-time intensivists (critical-care specialists), rather than relying on busy anaesthetists to also cover intensive care. This, he argued, would allow for children to be discharged from intensive care more quickly, thus freeing up beds.

His communication was referred to the Crumlin board, where it ruffled the feathers of colleagues opposed to the suggestion. 'It became a source of huge animosity, and something that later knocked over into the children's hospital debate. Life was made very difficult for me.'

Starved of government support, the children's health service became ever more dependent on donations to support new facilities. Parents' accommodation in Crumlin was funded with the proceeds of a *Late Late Show* appeal, while a new infectious diseases unit was built using the proceeds of a testimonial match for footballer Niall Quinn.

Professor Owen Smith, a haematologist in Crumlin, described conditions at the hospital as 'of eastern European standard'. The hospital would fail a hygiene test, he predicted, as patient care was being compromised 'across the board'.

While Crumlin and Temple Street were both agitating for

redevelopment, Dublin's third children's hospital, in Tallaght, was also unhappy with its lot.

Tallaght Hospital, following its long-overdue opening in 1998, included the old National Children's Hospital (NCH) formerly based in Harcourt Street. This amalgam of three very different hospitals – two with a Protestant ethos and one with a Catholic one; two adult hospitals and a children's one – endured a difficult start. 'It opened with a huge mortgage. Then services that were promised took a long time to arrive, and some never did,' says Triona Murphy, a long-standing member of the Tallaght Hospital Action Group.

The hospital endured controversies over patient safety and record-keeping in those early years, and eventually needed a large debt write-off from the HSE. Children's haematology moved to Crumlin. A promised obesity service failed to materialise, according to Murphy.

The hospital struggled to compete with more established rivals closer to the city centre. 'I could see how the population was expanding all around me and how people were worried about losing essential services,' Murphy, then a mother of three young children and a nurse in the hospital, says.

Tallaght was stuck in a chicken-and-egg situation. It wasn't attracting enough resources because it didn't have enough medical clout, yet it wouldn't get more clout until it got those extra resources. That might change if the hospital could persuade Crumlin to transfer to its campus. There was plenty of room there, and siting the new development promised by government where a children's service already existed made sense.

~

Brendan Drumm remembers, as he was growing up in County Leitrim, when his father was appointed manager of the local cooperative in Manorhamilton. It was on the point of financial collapse after improvements to the infrastructure for transporting milk led to smaller creameries being bypassed, rendering them financially unviable.

John Drumm felt the only way of saving the central co-op was to close five creameries in the area. This made him immensely unpopular, according to his son: 'Understandably so, given the village creamery was a focal point for farmers and therefore vital for local shops and pubs. But if he hadn't restructured, the co-op would have closed.'

The elder Drumm had also helped establish a secondary school in the village in the early 1970s. Unusually for the time and place, it was open to boys and girls, Catholics and Protestants. His son believes it is the only time a secondary school was established through a limited company. 'Creating it required a great capacity to be unpopular with various groups,' he says. 'The local Catholic hierarchy, for example, did all it could to frustrate the development of the new school.'

John Drumm, remembered by his son as 'a socialist who didn't believe in possessions', remained a huge influence on Brendan during his own career. 'He was constantly striving to improve things at a community level. Some of these projects were not universally popular and the criticism directed at him was embarrassing for us as children. Yet he provided constant reassurance, stressing that criticism from powerful interests was to be expected. *Achieving the ultimate goal was what mattered.*'

Drawing inspiration from his father, the Crumlin-based paediatrician thought nothing of highlighting the various turf wars between the children's hospitals, including his own, in pursuit of his ultimate goal of a single national children's hospital.

He has no regrets now about being so outspoken. The insistence of the three hospitals on maintaining separate services for paediatric surgery was 'unacceptable by international norms'. Leukaemia was being treated at two sites, despite small patient numbers, when it would make more sense to develop a single specialist centre. 'The situation was being sustained by the Department of Health, with successive governments refusing to challenge the powerful vested interests represented by the individual hospital boards.'

In 50 years, the boards of the three hospitals had never met to discuss bringing together services and optimising care for children, Drumm points out. 'That is frightening. And quite the opposite – they spent those years fighting one another over the location of specialist services. As a consequence, consultant posts in vital areas remained unfilled.'

In December 2003, Dublin planners gave the go-ahead for the redevelopment of the Mater adult hospital and the creation of a six-storey children's hospital on its campus to replace Temple Street. Still the government dithered over funding.

The general election of 2002 had returned a coalition of Fianna

Fáil and the pro-enterprise, socially liberal Progressive Democrats (PDs). Micheál Martin continued as minister for health. In March 2004, the measure for which he is best known, the workplace smoking ban, was introduced. Otherwise, Martin, whose predecessor Brian Cowen had nicknamed the department 'Angola' because of the number of landmine issues there that were waiting to blow up an unwary minister, endured a torrid time. He was criticised for commissioning dozens of reports into the structure and reform of the health service instead of making decisions.

Ultimately, he did oversee proposals to scrap the regional health boards running the health service and replace them with a new centralised and supposedly depoliticised body. But before it could be finalised, a government reshuffle in September 2004 saw him replaced by PD leader and tánaiste Mary Harney.

It therefore fell to Harney, a TD since 1981 and a minister since 1997, to see through the creation of the Health Service Executive. Henceforth, the role of the Department of Health was to be policy formation, while the HSE assumed responsibility for delivering services. The idea was to integrate health services centrally, and create a national point of responsibility for the problem-ridden sector. But with the new body absorbing all the staff in the old health boards, the HSE quickly became weighed down with bureaucracy after it was created in January 2005. Whenever something went wrong in the health service, the HSE was blamed.

Health reform was the PD's next major project, following the transformation of the tax system, according to Harney. The new minister vowed to deliver radical change, including the use of private investment to create much-needed health infrastructure.

'Hospitals are very expensive to build and equip and they could absorb every last euro available,' she warned, addressing her party conference in April 2005.

Bed shortages would be addressed by having private companies build hospitals on the grounds of existing public hospitals, Harney announced. One of the biggest proposals was for a 200-bed private hospital on the grounds of St James's. None of these projects was built, for a mixture of reasons, including political opposition, planning delays and the subsequent economic downturn. The plan for St James's Hospital got planning permission but was scrapped by a subsequent government. Years would pass before another facility, the national children's hospital, was proposed at the same location.

In her conference address, Harney singled out the replacement of Crumlin as one of her priorities, but suggested this could not be achieved promptly without additional private funding. 'How quickly can we do it? Parents just want the result, and not in ten years' time. But that too will mean change.'

But what kind of change? By now, alarm bells were ringing in government departments about the various plans in children's health. The proposed redevelopment of Crumlin could cost up to €500 million, according to one estimate. That would make it the most expensive healthcare project in the history of the state. And this was on top of the price tag for moving Temple Street to the Mater, then estimated to cost €400 million. And now there was talk of raising money privately.

'There was lots of handwringing about the plan for Crumlin,' says Karl Anderson. 'Yet things didn't change discernibly that I noticed. It wasn't moving any farther forward.'

Crumlin clearly required investment, but it was estimated that redevelopment would take 11 years due to the nature of the site and the need to maintain services during construction. Discussions about a possible move to other hospitals had petered out. Now opinion within the hospital was split between rebuilding on the site or switching to a greenfield location. Tallaght waited hopefully, a willing suitor.

Fate intervened to influence events. In September 2004, Professor Aidan Halligan had been appointed to run the HSE. A Dubliner who spent much of his working career in England, Halligan was at the time deputy chief medical officer in the UK and had been heavily involved in efforts to modernise Britain's National Health Service.

Two months later, he changed his mind, opting to stay with the NHS. Reports at the time diplomatically attributed his decision to family reasons. In fact, Halligan had told the government he needed sufficient powers to effect major changes to the health service, including the rationalisation of hospitals and staff. Ministers, spooked by the prospect of redundancies, baulked. Halligan backed out of the appointment and stayed in England.

His change of mind left the government in a hole. The HSE came into existence without a chief executive. One had to be found quickly. And who better to take over the running of the health service than Drumm, then aged 48 and heavily involved in various health-reform initiatives? Right place, right time, once again.

Still, there were hiccups. On several occasions, Drumm walked away from negotiations on the €400,000 a year job. A major sticking point was his insistence on appointing five external advisors from outside the HSE to help with strategic planning and change implementation. This was seen within the organisation as a vote of no-confidence in its senior executives.

The HSE board eventually approved the appointments sought by Drumm, but there was further disagreement over the provision of a consultant post for him after he finished his five-year term leading the health service.

It wasn't an auspicious start for the new organisation but Drumm got his way and, in August 2005, he was named as the first chief executive of the HSE. Henceforth, it was envisaged, politics would be taken out of decision-making around health services. The idea was to get away from the traditional local rivalries that had undermined reform in health and allow for difficult but necessary decisions to be taken, even if they were controversial.

Harney and Drumm would soon embark on a highly contested reform agenda, closing smaller emergency departments, centralising cancer services and cutting drug prices. Emulating his father, Drumm quickly developed the capacity to be unpopular with groups affected by his decisions and to plough on, regardless of opposition.

Something else was on the paediatrician's mind, now that he could influence the direction of health policy. 'The issue of a new children's hospital wasn't on anyone's agenda at this point,' he says. 'But when I was offered the post of CEO of the health service, I could see it represented a wonderful opportunity to reignite the idea and possibly even see it delivered.'

He wasn't interested in simply rebuilding Crumlin or

resurrecting Temple Street on the Mater site. His vision was to create a single, national institution, big enough to provide specialised treatment for the sickest children in the country under one roof. This wouldn't be any ordinary hospital; what he envisaged was the country's first mega-hospital.

'The thing about Brendan is, he was always ahead of everyone else in his strategic thinking,' one senior civil servant at the time observes.

Drumm hadn't intended to address the children's hospital issue immediately, but events forced his hand. The chaos around stalled hospital planning was reverberating across the health service. There was outrage in the midlands, for example, as the HSE put the redevelopment of Mullingar Hospital on hold, owing to the number of other projects in the pipeline.

By now, the rebuilding of Temple Street at the Mater was ready to go to tender after the proposal was confirmed by the HSE. When that happened, he realised, it would be impossible for the minister for health and the government not to proceed with the project.

'But the new hospital wasn't large enough. I was being asked to invest a huge tranche of public funds in a project that would never provide optimal care for sick children. We would be embedding the provision of specialist services for children across three sites for the next 50 years. I wasn't willing to do this. I believed the HSE board and the minister should also refuse to endorse the plan.'

Drumm sought to redirect policy – and quickly. The way to do this, he realised, was to get government to agree to the long-promised independent review of paediatric services. And to have this carried out by overseas experts, well removed from the hubbub of Irish medical politics.

The HSE board and the minister agreed to his proposal to appoint external consultants. In August, the same month Drumm took over at the HSE, Harney put the move of Temple Street to the Mater on hold.

'When I went into the Department of Health, the plan was to build a hospital for Temple Street and one for Crumlin,' Harney recalls. 'Nobody had ever really questioned that. Then Brendan came in to see me. He put the idea in my head by asking why were we planning to build two children's hospitals. And I thought, *Why are we building two?*'

Harney hadn't expressed any strong views on the issue up to this point, other than suggesting Crumlin be rebuilt at a different location. This still seemed to be her preferred option: 'It would take a lot longer to construct a new hospital on this site and it would also be very disruptive to the operation of the hospital if it was a construction site for a long number of years,' she told journalists in September 2005. Specialised treatment services for children should not be spread across 'a number of sites', she counselled, but this did not mean that three children's hospitals in Dublin were 'too many'.

The minister did favour the centralisation of specialised services for children – 'everybody agrees that tertiary facilities for sick children should be at a single location'. But, mindful perhaps of her boss Bertie Ahern's support for the Mater, she advised that general care facilities be maintained on each side of the city.

At the time, Harney was overseeing the controversial but ultimately successful centralisation of cancer services in eight centres, from over 30 previously. The guiding principle here was that treating more patients in the one place aided specialisation and resulted in better patient outcomes. As she explains to me when we talk 20 years on: 'All the international evidence is for [the link between] volume and quality.'

The decision to pause the move of Temple Street to the Mater provoked a furious outcry in both hospitals. Here was Drumm, a consultant who had worked in Crumlin, now head of the HSE, blocking the redevelopment of that hospital's main rival – or so it was viewed. Were Crumlin to move to Tallaght, for example, the resulting hospital on Dublin's southside would dwarf Temple Street.

In September, a month after his appointment, Drumm told the Oireachtas health committee that the new national children's hospital 'should ideally be in the city centre or close to the Mater site'.

To some, this sounded dangerously close to putting the cart before the horse. Had a decision been made about where to site the hospital before the promised independent review had taken place? Or was the HSE boss seeking to assuage bruised egos in Temple Street?

'This was simply a statement of fact,' Drumm tells me. 'Reassuring Temple Street was essential in view of the huge pressure that they were exerting on the political system to reverse the decision to stall their planned hospital.'

In the zero-sum game of medical politics, Crumlin welcomed the HSE's decision. Parents of children attending the hospital, still campaigning for new facilities, were also supportive. 'Temple

Street had to be stopped or kids would continue to fall between the cracks of different specialties,' says Linda Dillon. Henceforth, the parents would back whatever offered the best hope of a super-hospital, rather than the narrower interests of any single hospital.

Doctors in the city cleaved into opposing factions. 'We had paediatricians on the north side of the city saying that a single, specialised centre was not important for optimal children's care and yet the paediatricians on the south side of the city fully endorsed this as being necessary,' Drumm observes. 'The goal of providing optimal care for children was secondary to the parochial interests of the hospitals.'

Staff in Temple Street expressed shock at the last-minute decision to block the project. 'If the decision to call off the new Temple Street is not reversed, it will be a major lost opportunity for children,' 22 consultants warned in a letter to *The Irish Times* in January 2006. The 'sabotage' of the project illustrated 'all that is wrong with our health service'.

The letter still rankles with Drumm. 'As a paediatrician, it seemed particularly unfair to be accused by my professional colleagues of sabotage and of undermining the care of sick children.' But it was only a foretaste of the bitterness that was to come.

McKinsey & Co., a US management consultancy with huge experience of healthcare across the world, was engaged to examine the review. The firm was given just three months to complete its work. The terms of reference were general enough; the consultants were asked to decide whether tertiary services for children should in future be provided at 'one or more locations'.

However, not everyone felt the consultants were operating in a vacuum. 'When you hire somebody to do something, they'll ask you what you want to do in the first instance,' one close observer of the process tells me. 'The context here was the – well-founded – premise that there should be one paediatric hospital. But it was very contentious. The Mater was really opposed to it at first.'

'I would have queries about how the review was framed,' Triona Murphy says. 'If you ask the right question, you'll get the right answer.' While supportive of the proposal for a single tertiary hospital for children, she believed two secondary care centres were also needed, given the increase in population.

Irish health has seldom moved as fast as it did when the idea of a single national hospital for children first made it onto the political agenda. Largely, this is the result of one man's determination. Having found himself in the right place to influence events, Brendan Drumm had the focus to outthink other viewpoints and change the political narrative, while moving at such speed as to ensure that his work could not be undone.

'There's no doubt that Brendan was the driving force behind the single entity,' says Harney. 'But it made eminent sense. And all the international evidence was for it.'

7

Shock Waves and Discombobulation

'You cannot have two paediatric tertiary care centres focusing on different niches ... I challenge you to find me an example of where that works.'

The view of an unnamed overseas expert in children's medicine, quoted in the McKinsey report, *Children's Health First*

'I was ecstatic and I believed that most of my colleagues in health would also be.'

Brendan Drumm, describing his reaction to the decision by minister for health Mary Harney to give the go-ahead for a single national children's hospital in February 2006

The sun had long set and the streets had emptied as Brendan Drumm sat patiently in his car in Dublin city centre on the evening of 2 February 2006. High above him, on an upper floor of an office block, the fate of his plan for a single national children's hospital was being decided.

Hawkins House, a 12-storey block often described as Dublin's ugliest building (it was demolished in 2021), housed the offices of the minister for health and her officials. The adjacent car park in which Drumm waited was a wasteland of concrete and tarmac. No place to hang about on a bleak winter night, yet there was no option but to wait for white smoke.

The proposal for a single children's hospital was moving forward at breakneck speed. The McKinsey consultants completed their report backing the idea in five weeks. Drumm took it to the HSE board for approval within two days of receipt. On the same day, he briefed Mary Harney, before withdrawing to allow the civil servants and their minister to discuss options.

Harney had been sympathetic but she warned Drumm that it might be difficult to convince her officials to change tack from existing policy, which was to move Temple Street to the Mater. Nonetheless, that evening, she convened a snap meeting of senior civil servants to discuss the proposal.

At eight o'clock, Harney came down to him with an update. 'There was a lot of resistance,' he recalls. 'The officials wanted more time to consider the recommendations, she told me. This was a significant challenge for them, I understood that. They were not used to having to make up their minds in a couple of hours about a €500 million project, the largest ever capital commitment to an Irish healthcare project. They knew it was going to antagonise some.'

Drumm pleaded with the minister to persevere. If McKinsey wasn't accepted promptly, he warned, Temple Street would insist that its project proceed. The single hospital proposal in the report would be fatally undermined.

'The civil servants were saying, "Oh, minister, we'll have to take that report and study it. Let's not make any brave decisions here"', another source tells me. 'But she said, "No, we're going to publish it tomorrow."'

'I could appreciate how much pressure she was under,' Drumm says. 'It would have been so easy for her to say that she wanted to take more time. But she said she could see how important it was. She would go back up to the office and make the case.'

The text of the McKinsey report was explicit about the need for a single centre of excellence, and backed this up with forceful quotations from children's health experts arguing against the duplication of services. 'You cannot have two paediatric tertiary care centres focusing on different niches ... I challenge you to find me an example of where that works,' said one.

'We have two children's hospitals within two miles of each other,' said another. 'Neither of us is big enough to provide all the sub-specialties, and children need more than one sub-specialist, so it's hard to decide what to put where and what to share.'

'[We have] multiple hospitals [that] really struggle with critical mass,' according to a third, quoted in the report. 'How can you provide a service with one specialist? You cannot. He cannot be on call 24/7 and not have holidays.'

Each of these experts could have been describing the situation in Dublin, a city of modest size where children were being treated at three different locations.

But these lines from McKinsey's report, *Children's Health First*, were from doctors and hospital administrators outside Ireland, based in some of the leading children's hospitals in the world.

McKinsey had focused on best practice in children's healthcare in 15 countries, including Australia, Canada, Sweden, Norway, the UK, the US and New Zealand. Its consultants displayed no interest in the views of Irish paediatricians.

The 64-page report tracked the huge changes in the delivery of paediatric services over the preceding 40 years. No longer were sick children cared for alongside adults, but in specialised regional or national centres with large catchment areas. The bigger the children's hospital, the better the outcome, was the report's clear finding – whether in cardiac care, intensive care, oncology, organ transplants or anaesthetics. Multiple research papers were cited in support of this conclusion.

'The findings were broadly similar to the ones we reached back in 1993,' says paediatrician Gerry Loftus, 'but this was international and, therefore, it had more oomph.'

With an average catchment population of about three to five million, the world's best children's hospitals described in the report were able to offer a wider and deeper range of services. This evolution was driven by technological advances and a trend towards increased sub-specialisation. (By way of example, sub-specialties of paediatrics include paediatric cardiology and neonatal medicine.)

'Quality is critically dependent on having genuine breadth and depth in sub-specialist services – a "critical mass",' the authors of the report concluded.

One fact spoke louder in the report than any other. Of 17 hospitals examined by McKinsey, 15 were colocated with adult services. One was colocated with women's services only, and only one – Great Ormond Street in London – was entirely standalone.

Dublin should follow the example of other leading cities by creating a single new 'world-class tertiary centre' for children's health, the report recommended. This should 'ideally' be colocated with a leading adult academic hospital, in order to benefit from healthcare and academic linkages. The new hospital should have space for future expansion and be easily accessible by public transport and the road network.

Even McKinsey struggled with a definition of tertiary care. Depending on who the consultants talked to, 'tertiary' included 'complex kids' and 'anything that's referred from another doctor' to 'anything that could require ICU'. Even common conditions in patients with pre-existing diseases should be treated as tertiary cases, other doctors asserted. Ultimately, the report adopted a broad definition of tertiary cases based on diagnosis, rather than where children were treated, saying, 'Whether a case is secondary or tertiary is a clinical judgement, which will vary by physician.'

'What people don't understand about a tertiary hospital is that it's not for the falls off swings, the broken arms, that kind of stuff,' says Brian Gilroy, an engineer who was appointed head of estates in the HSE at this time, responsible for managing the organisation's property portfolio and capital development. 'That's secondary care and you can get that anywhere. Tertiary is the medicine that you can't get anywhere else in the country.'

A lack of precision over the meaning of tertiary services persisted through the subsequent debate on the children's hospital, as McKinsey's central recommendation of colocation of children's services with an adult hospital got lost in a fog of alternative suggestions – most notably, that it be colocated with a maternity hospital rather than an adult one. Moreover, allowing doctors to apply their own definition of 'tertiary' medicine, as suggested by McKinsey, exposed those designing the hospital later to increased demands for space and other resources.

The report attempted to forecast future demand for a single children's hospital, linking it not just to the overall population growth rate, but also to expectations of shifts of population within the country and 'moderate' international immigration up to 2020.

Its estimates, based on figures from the Central Statistics Office (CSO), would prove reasonably accurate. Immigration rose sharply in the decades after 2006, apart from the years after the economic crash. Ireland's population grew by 17 per cent between 2006 and 2020, and by about 25 per cent to 2025. Falling birth rates offset the impact of immigration in younger age groups. In 2024, the CSO reported that the population aged 0–14 was 1.01 million, close to McKinsey's 2006 estimate for 2021 of 1.016 million.

Based on this analysis of future demand, the report recommended a single tertiary centre with 380 regular, intensive-care and day beds. Of this total, 230 of these should be for secondary care in the greater Dublin area and the remainder for tertiary care beds for the entire country. This was big, but not so big as to rank in the top ten largest children's hospitals in the US.

Drumm continued to linger in the car park below Hawkins House like an expectant father, anxiously awaiting news. Thirteen years after he and other paediatricians had first nurtured the idea of a single national children's hospital, a political decision seemed imminent.

Harney reappeared in the gloom shortly before nine o'clock with the decision he was hoping for. 'There was agreement. She would bring the proposal to government for endorsement.'

The die was cast. Ireland would build a single new children's hospital, and it would be located alongside an adult hospital. 'That decision completely changed the dynamic, there and then,' Karl Anderson says. 'The argument moved from "should" to "how".'

The plan was announced the following day, 3 February 2006, at a press conference attended by parent groups and children's hospital representatives. The site would be chosen by a group of public servants.

'I was ecstatic,' Drumm says, 'and I believed that most of my colleagues in health would also be.'

However, the McKinsey report sent shock waves through Dublin medical circles. Up to this point, the debate had been about renovating existing institutions, and where to provide the most complex treatments for children – heart operations, for example. There was general agreement that specialised services needed to be consolidated on individual sites, but it was expected that different specialties might end up in different hospitals.

Just a few months before, Harney had been saying there was still room in the capital for more than one children's hospital. Now the plan was to provide almost all specialised services for children on one site. The exception was local emergency services, but even here, there would be no overnight beds at other locations in Dublin. This was consolidation of services on a level not seen before in Irish health.

In case anyone wasn't clear on the implications, Drumm spelled them out on publication of the report. The plan meant an end to Crumlin hospital as it then existed, he said. The new hospital would be sited alongside an adult hospital, so there would be no rebuilding at Crumlin. As for Temple Street and the children's hospital in Tallaght, they would close unless they won the competition to build the new hospital.

The HSE boss cautioned against any assumption that the new hospital would be sited at either the Mater, to which Temple Street had been due to move, or Tallaght. 'I'm sure there are other adult facilities in this city who will want to be considered in the process,' he said.

The recommendation for colocating a children's hospital with an adult one represented a major change from previous policy, which was to consolidate specialist services for children in different locations. Even Drumm admits that, at first, he wasn't in favour since he feared a children's hospital would be 'buried' by the much larger adult facility.

The report was relatively well received on the day it was announced. Temple Street welcomed its emphasis on colocation with an adult hospital, which had the happy consequence of ruling out rivals that lacked an on-site tertiary adult hospital. Tallaght didn't comment but its chief executive had already expressed support for colocation with an adult hospital. Crumlin merely said it was committed to working with the taskforce being set up to decide where centralised services should be located.

Just a week earlier, Temple Street doctors had been accusing the HSE and government of sabotaging its move to the Mater. Now one of the authors of that letter was reported as saying that there was 'a lot more' in the review than he had expected.

'By opening the door to adult teaching hospitals instead of just the three children's hospitals in Dublin located at Temple Street, Crumlin and Tallaght, previous strategies for the development of paediatric services in Ireland were thrown into disarray,' *The Irish Times* commented on the day after the announcement. 'The real battle may only be starting' as rival hospitals vie to win the project, its health correspondent Eithne Donnellan presciently observed.

Alternative views were expressed as the reality of the proposals sank in. Crumlin said it favoured colocation with both an adult and a maternity hospital. In March, a patient group, Children in Hospital Ireland, expressed concern over the proposed colocation with an adult hospital. Why not care for children in a standalone facility, a major academic teaching hospital in its own right, asked its chief executive, Mary O'Connor.

In politics, discombobulation was the order of the day. Politicians from opposition parties were wary of being seen to go against a project as transparently virtuous as a children's hospital. According to Labour leader Pat Rabbitte, the merits of the report were accepted but 'many people were a little bemused at the policy priority being given to this'.

Talk inevitably turned to who might win the project. St James's, arguably the Mater's main rival, had just come through a busy few years developing new facilities on its campus, leading some observers to believe the country's biggest hospital wouldn't be interested (wrongly, as it turned out). 'Everything was pointing to the Mater being the chosen site by this stage,' one closely placed source maintains.

Insofar as cost was an issue at this point, it related to the millions of euro already spent on the plan to move Temple Street as part of the Mater redevelopment. Although Drumm claimed this was not wasted money, that might depend on where the project was sited. The new hospital could be built for 'an awful lot less' than the estimated cost of moving Temple Street and rebuilding Crumlin, he promised.

It had been decided to build an Irish 'super-hospital' for children, and discussions and debate had begun about its location. But who would make this decision?

The consultants had finished their work. Perhaps it was a mistake not to have given the job of selecting the site for the new hospital to these outsiders, who were more likely to be seen as impartial. 'Mary Harney should have asked McKinsey to determine where the hospital should go,' Louis Roden believes.

'Maybe in hindsight we should have done that,' says Harney. 'But I never for a minute thought the site would become such an issue. Not once we had the evidence that this was the way to go. And even if McKinsey had picked the site, I don't think it would have made any difference to the opposition. It was so vicious.'

A site could only be chosen *after* a decision was made to colocate the children's hospital with an adult one, Drumm maintains. 'We couldn't spend money on siting the hospital in a particular location until the McKinsey recommendations [on colocation] were available and accepted by the HSE and government. Then we had a very short time to review potential sites, because of the hold that had been put on Temple Street's redevelopment and the public pressure being exerted on behalf of the hospital.'

Accordingly, the job of advising on the optimum location for the hospital was handed to a 'task group' composed of low-profile officials from the HSE, Department of Health and Office of Public Works. Ultimately, the decision would be taken by government.

The stakes were huge, and all the main Dublin hospitals knew it. The winners of this contest would benefit from the biggest project in Irish healthcare. Resources would flow to their hospital for years to come, and prestige would follow. Cutting-edge medicine for children would end up being concentrated there. Their opportunities for private medicine would multiply, in both the adult and the colocated children's hospital. In contrast, the losers risked decades of relative neglect, as their hospitals slipped down the list of official priorities.

With a general election looming, government candidates in parts of Dublin faced a hammering if the decision looked as if it was going against local interests. Bertie Ahern in particular would lose face if he was unable to land such a big project for the Mater, in his constituency. Northsiders were already complaining on radio chat-shows about the possibility of having to cross the Liffey to bring their child to hospital (oblivious to the fact that parents of sick children across Ireland have much farther to travel).

And a new element entered the mix, with a variety of private business consortiums offering to build the hospital in locations well removed from an existing healthcare setting. It seemed no one was paying heed to the McKinsey recommendations and nearly everyone had a back field where a children's hospital could be built.

In all, 22 locations were suggested by their owners to the task group. As well as the six Dublin teaching hospitals, the list included Mountjoy Prison, a golf club in west Dublin and a psychiatric hospital in the north of the county.

Most of the Dublin adult teaching hospitals wanted to host the new hospital. Tallaght highlighted the space available on its campus and its nearby Luas stop, but it was never regarded as a frontrunner. 'Our chances were slim,' Triona Murphy recalls. 'It was down to medical politics, which can be even more extreme than regular politics. I don't think there was enough firepower on campus to fight for us.'

Connolly Hospital in Blanchardstown, which had been founded as a tuberculosis sanatorium in 1955 and repurposed as a general hospital in 1973, also applied to host the project. Though small, its strengths included adequate space and a location beside the M50 motorway. Beaumont Hospital highlighted its expertise in neurology and kidney transplantation. The private-sector Beacon Medical Group suggested building the facility alongside an as yet unopened adult hospital in Sandyford, and having it run by St Vincent's Hospital.

One proposal suggested merging Crumlin and the Coombe, a maternity and women's hospital dating back to the early nineteenth century, on a site near the South Circular Road in Dublin. Amalgamating the children's facilities in Crumlin and Tallaght in the latter location was also proposed.

Solicitor and property developer Noel Smyth emerged as the frontrunner among the private proposals. A media-savvy figure frequently in the public eye, Smyth was best known for his legal representation of former supermarket tycoon Ben Dunne. Working on a case for Dunne against his family trust, Smyth had uncovered €1.3 million in payments his client had made to former taoiseach Charles Haughey. The solicitor's evidence at a subsequent tribunal helped seal Haughey's late-life humiliation.

Smyth was friendly with consultants in Crumlin and had served for a time on the hospital board, so he was familiar with its infrastructure problems. To address these, he developed a proposal to site the planned new children's hospital on a 32-acre greenfield plot at Newlands Cross, near the M50, backed by a consortium of banks and construction firms. The building would be standalone, with Tallaght Hospital a mile away. It would be self-financing, Smyth envisaged, by charging the state for services on a 'per item' basis. Crumlin hospital wasn't owned by the state, he pointed out, and neither would the new facility he was planning (ownership would rest with an independent foundation).

The plan gained currency on radio chat shows, though McKinsey's recommendation for colocation with an adult hospital was frequently overlooked. However, it failed to gain political traction. Officialdom had its report and its ministerial decision, envisaging a different direction of travel. Mary Harney was unenthusiastic, despite Smyth's site being in her constituency, given the seeming lack of state control over running costs. 'This proposal would have involved the state writing a blank cheque for the project, through a fee-for-service arrangement,' she says.

The task group was initially given two months to come to a decision. This was extended to allow consideration of the proposals from the private sector, and to assess whether the new hospital should include a maternity hospital or unit.

In the end, the group didn't feel it had the time or scope to decide on the future configuration of maternity services but it did recommend that the winning site should be able to show it also had the space for these services.

The winners would have to make the site available to the HSE unencumbered, the group decided. 'That was regarded as critical, even if the HSE was never going to be operating the hospital,' one of those involved in the selection process tells me. Effectively, this recommendation spared the children's hospital the kinds of argument over ethos that have plagued subsequent projects, such as the move of the National Maternity Hospital to St Vincent's Hospital campus.

The winning location would have to show that its adult hospital offered a broad range of specialties, according to a second key criterion set by the task group. This made St James's and the Mater clear favourites, thanks to the 'womb to tomb' care they provided on their campuses.

Both hospitals enjoyed enthusiastic academic backing – St James's from Trinity College and the Mater from UCD (whose president, Hugh Brady, was a medical professor). Hospitals are vital for university medical schools because they provide training spaces for students and interns. The bigger the hospital, the more medical students a college can recruit.

Yet both St James's and the Mater lacked space. Access and traffic were also issues, though the Luas ran by St James's and, at the time, a metro was planned that would pass under the Mater.

Amid the competing claims, there was little media or political focus on cost. The bar had already been set high by McKinsey, which had benchmarked Dublin against the finest children's hospitals in the world. What was good enough for London, Stockholm, Toronto or Houston was good enough for Ireland.

'It was 2006–7, the height of the Celtic Tiger. There was a huge amount of hubris around,' Gerry Loftus says. 'People were saying, "We have one chance to get it right", so they went all in. It was: "This is a once-in-a-generation chance." Everything just ballooned after that.'

8

Magical Thinking and the Mater

'It really didn't matter where you put the children's hospital, so long as it was beside St James's or the Mater. Between the two of them, it was six of one, half dozen of the other.'

Brian Gilroy, former head of estates, HSE

'I didn't give a damn where I brought my child so long as the best treatment was there.'

Louis Roden of the New Crumlin Hospital Group

Dublin buzzed with rumours as 2006 dragged on and the task group's deliberations continued. Depending on whom you talked to, the children's hospital was a 'stitch-up' for the Mater, it was going to land beside St James's Hospital, or it was destined for a greenfield site in west Dublin, either adjacent to Tallaght Hospital or elsewhere along the M50 motorway.

Working behind closed doors, the task group stuck to the criteria outlined in the McKinsey report. This group of Irish civil servants was not briefed to set aside the recommendations of the international experts, and neither was it going to do this of its own volition.

The private offers of land, while still featuring prominently in media coverage, were ruled out quickly because they were not adjacent to an adult hospital. Among the city's public teaching hospitals, Tallaght Hospital, St Vincent's Hospital and Connolly Hospital in Blanchardstown were next to be excluded because they had fewer consultants and less clinical specialisation than the biggest facilities.

That left three institutions in the running – the Mater, St James's and Beaumont. But Beaumont, located deep in a north Dublin housing estate, was judged to be 'significantly less suitable' in terms of access.

The choice therefore lay between the two biggest adult hospitals in the city – the Mater and St James's. But a problem had already arisen – the chairman of the task group, John O'Brien, was a former chief executive of St James's. O'Brien had to step down in April and was replaced by another HSE official, Laverne McGuinness.

The task group, all public servants and no medics, wasn't able to distinguish between the bids from the Mater and St James's on grounds of clinical strengths, planning issues, access and governance. But both hospitals were found to have sufficient room for a children's hospital and a maternity hospital.

The group then took an extraordinary decision. At this late stage of deliberations, in May 2006, members decided to add two further criteria on which a final choice would be made. The first was timescale – how soon a hospital could be built. The second related to maximising access to medical specialties in other adult hospitals around Dublin.

A children's hospital could be completed more quickly at the Mater, the group determined, because significant work had already been done in preparation for the move of Temple Street to that site. And the Mater site, because it was situated marginally closer to other hospitals than St James's, was considered to be better placed to call in specialist expertise – such as neurosurgery or transplantation in Beaumont – from them.

The Mater got the nod, by a hair's breadth. It did so, not because it was a better fit for the project than St James's, but because some preparatory work had been done there for a smaller children's hospital than the one now envisaged.

Further details that might have influenced the task force's decision emerged from an academic thesis completed in 2007 by a former HSE executive, Phil Shovlin. During her research, Shovlin unearthed an internal document from Temple Street, *Further Configuration of Tertiary Paediatric Services in Ireland*, which suggested the development of a single national children's hospital at the Mater. But this document was dated May 2005, nine months before McKinsey published its report. It seems at this early stage that Temple Street wasn't just looking for a new children's hospital; it was already looking for *the* children's hospital.

Shovlin argues this proposal 'anchored' the decision-making process by the task group, which was hearing from advocacy groups that the hospital needed to be delivered quickly. She adds: 'The proposals within this document [from Temple Street] determined the decision outcome.'

The group had worked its way through scoring the original criteria, but had ended up with a 'dead heat', according to one member interviewed in the thesis. It still needed to differentiate between the bids from St James's and the Mater, but didn't have any medical members to turn to for advice. One member described the lack of a paediatrician on the task group as a deficit. Another told Shovlin that 'we didn't draw on them as a source of expertise ... because we did not think they could be particularly neutral about a site'.

Failing to make a clear decision – by giving an 'either/or' option – would probably be worse than no decision at all. The issue would simply end up as a political football, members realised. So, at a late stage, they added the two new criteria. It is hard to argue with Shovlin's conclusion that the result was a 'non-rational escalation of commitment to one hospital over another'.

The HSE board adopted the task group's report recommending the Mater in June 2006. The news had already leaked by the time the minister made the formal announcement, promising to build a 'multi-denominational and pluralist' children's hospital there. Her officials were tasked with preparing a formal case for the hospital for government approval.

There were no immediate costs to the Exchequer, according to Harney's memorandum to government, which I obtained under freedom of information legislation. The decision to proceed with a single 'super-hospital' for children 'is expected to prove less costly than previous plans' to redevelop both Crumlin and Temple Street (variously estimated to cost €700–900 million), the memorandum optimistically asserted.

The decision wasn't a surprise, but pushback against it was immediate and forceful. Now that a site had been identified, the backers of every other proposal ganged up on it.

Task group members had been told not to talk to the media. There seemed to be no communication strategy for the decision. 'Having made our announcement [we] effectively handed the playing field over to those who disagreed with the decision,' according to one member interviewed by Shovlin.

St James's described the process used to reach a decision as flawed and claimed that the Mater campus was too small and more inaccessible by car than its hospital. Professor Tom Mitchell, chairman of the St James's board and a former provost of Trinity College Dublin, accused the task force of 'clearly and egregiously' failing in its task by not taking greater account of the range of medical specialties available in the two hospitals.

As the largest hospital in the state, St James's boasted the largest number of consultants and specialties, it was true, though the Mater wasn't far behind. According to the task group report, St James's had 121 whole-time equivalent consultant posts, Beaumont had 110 and the Mater had 94. St James's was strong on blood disorders, burns and cancer; the Mater's strengths lay in heart medicine, spinal injuries and lung transplants.

Overnight, the stances of individual children's hospitals reversed. Staff at Crumlin, who had been enthusiastic about the task group process, now denounced it as failing to consult with paediatricians or parents. The report lacked detail and transparency, the hospital claimed.

Over at Temple Street, the previous downright opposition of its paediatricians converted into giddy support. Temple Street was getting its hospital at the Mater, and it would be even bigger than originally planned.

The decision meant that Tallaght had not only missed out on the big prize, but would also lose its existing children's hospital. On the streets of the suburb, more than 4,000 people demonstrated on a Saturday afternoon that autumn, calling for the creation of two children's hospitals, one on the northside and one next to the local adult hospital, on the southside.

The airwaves continued to teem with calls for the hospital to be built on the fringes of Dublin, along the M50, for the benefit of those living outside the city. In Ireland, the delineation between 'city' and 'country' is sharply drawn; debates about resources are often framed as 'Dublin versus the rest'. A proxy for this argument is often 'car' versus 'public transport'. The new hospital, a national institution serving the entire country, was always going to be located in Dublin, where the bulk of the population, and medical resources and training, are concentrated. But this part of the debate came to be about *how much* of a 'city project' the hospital would be, and the importance of access – vehicle access – relative to other issues. Time and again over the years that followed, the inner-city Mater proposition would be compared unfavourably with proposals to locate the hospital to the west of the city, which was more easily accessible by car from 'rural Ireland'.

The job of getting the project started fell to Brian Gilroy, the plain-spoken engineer who was head of estates at the HSE. From Dublin, Gilroy had spent most of his career working in the private sector before joining the new health body in 2006 to kick-start an ambitious new building programme.

The switch involved a change of culture, but Gilroy, a brother of the Dublin GAA player and manager Pat Gilroy, was happy to embrace the challenge. 'The public sector doesn't have to be a laggard, but you have to change the rules to get it to work,' he observes. 'That informed a lot of what I did. I tried innovative things. I had to be willing to fail. If an idea worked, people got on board.'

Charged with renewing the country's health infrastructure, Gilroy was initially sceptical about the plan for a new super-hospital. 'Why are we doing it the way we are doing it?' he remembers asking Drumm of the plan for a single children's hospital at the Mater. Drumm sent him on an information-gathering trip to North America to visit children's hospitals there.

In Toronto, he watched surgeons remove a tumour from the brain of a newborn, operating in real time with computer-guided equipment and using special ceramic instruments. Back in Ireland, doctors would have had to wait six months until the baby's organs had grown and they would be relying on scans put up on the wall of the operating theatre.

'I saw that you had to be doing a particular procedure every day; otherwise, you don't become proficient. And, for that, you need numbers. You have to colocate. That experience sold it to me.'

Arguments about the location of the hospital were to rage for years, from the moment a particular place was chosen. What side people took might be influenced by their medical affiliations, views on public versus private transport and their opinion on state versus private development.

'There was a lot of bullshit politics around this,' says Gilroy. 'It really didn't matter where you put the children's hospital, so long as it was beside St James's or the Mater. Between the two of them, it was six of one, half-dozen of the other.

'Putting a children's hospital on the outskirts of a city is a disaster,' he argues. 'You never get a break there if you're a parent. Put the hospital on a field by the M50 and parents are never going to get out of the place. There are no facilities around, just fields.

'Forget about building on the M50 unless the state is prepared to put a proper adult hospital there, and there wasn't – and isn't – the money for that,' is his blunt assessment.

For Drumm, the location was unimportant. Drawing on his father's approach to life, he believed what mattered was the ultimate goal – in this case, building a single national hospital for the sickest children. But at least the decision in favour of the Mater meant that he couldn't be accused of favouring his alma mater, Crumlin.

'I felt that whatever location was picked, it was going to have inadequacies. No site was going to be perfect. The critical thing was to make a decision and move on as quickly as possible. If we didn't, there was a huge risk of the government walking away.'

The government took its time about confirming the HSE recommendation. While ministers dithered, the arguments against the Mater came thick and fast, and they paid little heed to the criteria featuring in McKinsey and the other reports. By now familiar points were made, alleging a lack of space and access at the hospital.

In the media, private developers continued to pop up offering lands for a hospital, or even to build the hospital itself. 'Somebody seems to have identified in their mind some magical site in Dublin that we can all get free access to and we can all drive there in 20 minutes in the morning or evening, but nobody has actually come forward to identify this site,' a clearly frustrated Drumm complained on *The Marian Finucane Show* on RTÉ Radio 1 in January 2007.

Arguments about traffic and access to the Mater were a 'figment', he maintained. 'Looking across the world to centres in Toronto, Boston, Philadelphia, Birmingham, London – they're all in city-centre locations.'

If anything, opposition to the Mater hardened, driven by sympathetic coverage on radio chat shows and in newspaper opinion columns. For prominent political commentator Fintan O'Toole, the decision to site the hospital 'in a high-rise tower in the centre of Dublin City' at the Mater was 'a prime example of everything that is wrong with public governance in Ireland'. O'Toole followed others in alleging a lack of consultation with stakeholders and a lack of space that would necessitate the building of an 11-storey hospital.

A mini-controversy blew up over the extent of the task group's consultation with international medical experts. The doctors contacted were never asked their thoughts on individual sites, it emerged; their advice was sought on clinical issues alone. Journalists tracked down one eminent British professor who described his involvement with the task group as 'minimal' – just a brief phone call from an Irish civil servant.

The board of Crumlin rejoined the fray, also claiming the Mater site was too small and inaccessible, with too few parking spaces. There was insufficient space for a colocated maternity hospital, further expansion or even playgrounds, its representatives claimed. (Never mind that the playground in Crumlin had been demolished because so few children were using it.)

There would be no natural light on the first five storeys of the children's hospital on the Mater site, Geraldine Regan, Crumlin's director of nursing, claimed: 'Research has shown that sick children respond better to treatment where they have access to natural light and a pleasant outdoor environment.' Almost in vain, the HSE pointed out that the hospital had yet to be designed, so allegations of insufficient space and light were, at best, premature.

Crumlin, backed by opposition political parties, demanded an international peer-review group re-examine the plan and said it was prepared to accept a move to the Mater if this was the recommendation of the review.

Harney stood her ground: 'The people that advised on the location of the hospital were architects, engineers, the Office of

Public Works and experts from Trinity College. They recommended the site. I didn't, the HSE didn't.'

She wanted to get away from reviews, she told reporters. 'I do not believe it is in anyone's interest to delay and have more reviews. This hospital was never going to be located on a greenfield site. It needed to be colocated with an adult teaching hospital.'

That left Crumlin in a difficult position. Staff were overwhelmingly against merging with Temple Street as part of a new national children's hospital, but what were they *for*? Some didn't want to budge, while those who favoured a move had differing views on where the hospital should go.

The parents' group in Crumlin, meanwhile, backed the Mater proposal. 'I didn't care where the hospital was built,' says Linda Dillon. 'If you have a seriously ill child, you will get to wherever it is, and you'll be very glad that it's there. The taxi men and the letter-writers all had a view that it was in the wrong place. That had nothing to do with the [experience of] parents.'

Louis Roden makes a similar point: 'It seemed that everyone had a better idea than everyone else. But I didn't give a damn where I brought my child so long as the best treatment was there. The people with opinions weren't dealing with dying children. They weren't sleeping on the floor of Crumlin for six months.'

'The fear in the hospital was that it would be subsumed into Temple Street, that it would disappear,' Karl Anderson says. 'The idea that a new, independent, non-aligned hospital was being created just didn't get across.' Still, it seemed that the decision on a location for the project had been made, and would not be undone.

~

Given the history of territorialism in Irish medicine, opposition to the Mater plan was to be expected. Going back to the Mother and Child controversy in the 1950s and even earlier, issues around sick children have raised strong emotions. However, the vehemence with which the children's hospital project was being criticised was extraordinary.

The atmosphere around the decision-making process was febrile. 'Of all the issues I dealt with, including the reorganisation of cancer services, this was by far the most political and bitter,' Harney says of this period. 'The rivalry between the various institutions was unbelievable.

'The things that were said, the personal attacks, the undermining behind the scenes, it was just vicious, against Brendan Drumm and others. It was all about the individuals and not about the children. It really was an eye-opener for me.'

'The medical politics dictated everything,' says Bertie Ahern. 'It became a northside versus southside battle, driven by consultants and their friends in the media. The Crumlin guys were never off the radio. Southside was linked to Trinity College and keeping the liberal viewpoint. Northside was linked to UCD, and this was the Catholic view. Yet all that was only in the heads of a few yobbos on either side.'

Drumm received a series of abusive letters, unsigned, and a few signed ones too. Fearful that the project was being undermined by the arguments raging over its location, he cast around for alternative options. At the time, the HSE was transferring ownership of a 70-acre site at Grangegorman, north of Dublin's city centre, to the Dublin Institute of Technology (now Technological University Dublin) for a new campus. Why not build a new Mater Hospital and a new children's hospital side by side in Grangegorman?

There seemed to be enough land there to advance both the educational and health infrastructures, with scope for synergy between the two. Drumm floated the idea with Harney. On a quiet Sunday, he walked the land with Gerry Howlin, an advisor to Ahern who lived locally. Both were receptive.

However, the plan was going nowhere unless it had the support of the Mater. It, like many of the other hospitals in this story, was a voluntary institution – private but non-profit; independent despite being entirely state-funded.

The board of the hospital feared that the Grangegorman proposal might halt the onsite redevelopment that had been promised for so long. Even if it agreed to the proposal, it might never happen.

Ultimately, Drumm and the chairman of the Mater board went to meet the superior of the Sisters of Mercy, who owned the hospital, in Naas.

The nuns weren't interested. 'Unfortunately I couldn't convince the leadership of the order or the Mater board that this represented a unique opportunity to develop a great centre of excellence,' Drumm says. 'To this day, I regret this as a major missed opportunity for Irish healthcare.'

Drumm was the head of the health service, yet the decision here was the nuns' to make because the Mater was a voluntary hospital and they owned it. 'It emphasised the remarkable power that is vested in voluntary hospitals, allowing them to veto developments in the healthcare sector that the HSE and the government consider to be the best option for the country,' he observes. 'It was the same as the power being exerted by the individual children's hospitals in trying to determine how the new hospital would be developed to suit their own interests.'

Religion raised its head in the debate with a surprising new line of attack on the children's hospital plan, one that threatened to embarrass the government at a sensitive time in relations with Northern Ireland. The Good Friday Agreement had been signed less than a decade before and the IRA had laid down its arms only a year earlier, in July 2005.

Tallaght Hospital was a relatively new hospital fused out of three older hospitals with largely Protestant roots. Now the National Children's Hospital there was to be merged with two Catholic children's hospitals (Crumlin and Temple Street) and the resulting entity was to be located at another Catholic hospital, the Mater. Church of Ireland leaders were unhappy. Moving children's services out of Tallaght, they claimed, would breach that hospital's charter.

Never mind that the new children's hospital would be an independent, secular institution. The Mater had confirmed in writing to the task group review that it would cede the land needed for the new hospital, which would have its own board of management. The nuns later sought, and obtained, the requisite permission for this from Rome.

'I'm very seriously concerned about what is good for children,' the Church of Ireland archbishop of Dublin, John Neill, told *Magill* magazine. He recited now familiar arguments about a lack of space and poor transport links before getting to his point: 'I'm also concerned that the variety provided by the various hospitals and traditions [in Tallaght] is going to be lost and the ethos as it's reflected by the ethical approach of the hospital, and more liberal approaches described as Protestant.'

Neill specifically referred to issues relating to medical ethics, such as embryo treatment and genetics. He may have had in mind a controversial decision taken by the Mater's ethics committee in 2005, when it ruled that female cancer patients could not avail of a new trial drug because it required them to take the contraceptive pill.

The row had perhaps more to do with Tallaght itself than the children's hospital plan. Since it opened in 1998, Tallaght had been feeling neglected relative to other hospitals. Church of Ireland clergyman Dr Gordon Linney claimed it had been 'asset-stripped' by an uncaring HSE. 'There is a huge anti-Tallaght attitude. By not retaining a paediatric service at the Tallaght site, the government is walking away from a solemn commitment made by the entire Oireachtas [to keep the hospital's charter],' Linney, a member of the hospital's board, told *Magill*.

Worse than that, as Triona Murphy recalls, it was being 'left with nothing' following the decision to site all children's services at the Mater.

Not everyone within the Church of Ireland agreed that the hospital's charter was being breached. The dean of St Patrick's

Cathedral, Robert McCarthy, accused the archbishop of setting out to 'play the Protestant card' to secure the new hospital for Tallaght.

HSE chief executive Brendan Drumm pleaded for the decision about the new hospital to be made on medical rather than theological grounds. Yet opposition continued to mount. Church of Ireland leaders demanded a face-to-face meeting with the taoiseach.

In June 2006, they met Ahern, Harney, Drumm and senior civil servants in Government Buildings. Archbishop of Armagh Robin Eames warned the politicians that the transfer of children's services from Tallaght could potentially undermine the Northern Ireland peace agreement.

'People on our side of the table were astonished,' Drumm recalls of this claim. 'They probably believed the commitments made to them at the time Tallaght was founded were being contravened. But it would have been difficult to justify these commitments over international expert advice on what was best for Irish children.'

'We wanted to make sure the new hospital was controlled by the government, not the Catholic Church,' Linney tells me. 'And we wanted doctors to be free to prescribe what was best for the child. These were things we needed reassurance on.'

'I think we were able to satisfy them that this would not be a Catholic hospital or anything like that,' Harney tells me.

'There were no problems with the churches,' Ahern says. 'I got on well with Eames; he was easy with this stuff. Tallaght was worried that it mightn't hold its ethos in the new setup, but the nuns in the

Mater had given over the whole site to the state for the children's hospital.'

Ahern, a dab hand at negotiation, followed up the meeting with a letter giving assurances on Tallaght's status and promising a review of the hospital's funding. In time, a decision would be made to locate an urgent-care centre for children there. This strand of the opposition to the Mater proposal had been defused.

Other doubts were harder to expunge. Throughout this period, and long after it, critics of the Mater plan muttered darkly about the influence of Bertie Ahern in the decision. Official denials and a lack of evidence did nothing to dent claims of political interference.

An unrivalled vote-getter who became a three-term taoiseach, Ahern was long steeped in mystery and intrigue. The corrupt former taoiseach Charles Haughey, his mentor in politics, once described him as 'the most skilful, the most devious, the most cunning of them all'. Ahern was 'the most enigmatic leader ever chosen by Fianna Fáil, a paradox on every level', according to political journalist Stephen Collins in *The Power Game: Ireland under Fianna Fáil*.

Ahern's personal finances had long been the subject of scrutiny; as minister for finance in the 1990s, he didn't even have an active bank account. One of the few figures in public life identifiable by a first name only, his political style endlessly frustrated opponents, one of whom once described it as 'like playing handball against a haystack. You hear a dull thud but the ball never comes back to you'.

As the children's hospital was being proposed, Ahern was under investigation by a tribunal over payments from developers. Just a few years earlier, he had promoted the building of a 65,000-seater sports stadium in west Dublin, a project that was quickly dubbed the 'Bertie Bowl'.

The stadium never saw the light of day, due to cost fears and trenchant opposition. 'Over my dead body, I decided, would there be a Bertie Bowl before a much-needed children's hospital,' Linda Dillon, who at this time was spending long hours with her sick daughter in Crumlin, remembers thinking.

Was the new children's hospital, now to be located alongside the Mater in the taoiseach's constituency, another attempt to create a lasting political legacy? Had Ahern in some way influenced the decision?

Always avowedly in favour of plans to redevelop the Mater itself, Ahern has repeatedly denied any involvement in the decisions that led to the national children's hospital heading there. He even said he had 'misgivings' about this project going to the Mater.

'Bertie was furious' when the children's hospital was awarded to the Mater, says Harney. 'He thought it would delay the Mater [adult hospital redevelopment]. He actually told me he wasn't happy. I do believe him. I believe it was an honest process.'

'Bertie and I were accused in the media of having met to discuss his wish for the hospital to be based on the Mater site. This was untrue,' Drumm tells me. 'The taoiseach discussed the children's hospital development with me on only one occasion and that was to raise a concern that the decision on where it would be sited was delaying a planned major extension of the Mater adult hospital.'

Drumm is adamant that there was no interference in the process. 'No politician spoke to me about where the hospital should be located and I never met with the group tasked with choosing the site.'

Yet the controversy refused to go away. In the Dáil, Labour's Pat Rabbitte pointed to comments made by Des Lamont, chairman of the Mater, in September 2005, thanking the taoiseach for pledging the children's hospital to the Mater. This was before McKinsey was appointed and the task group made its recommendation.

Fine Gael senator Brian Hayes reached back even farther, quoting from a 2002 letter to then minister for health Micheál Martin. Ahern wrote: 'Given that the intention is to move Temple Street on to the Mater campus and to provide a state-of-the-art children's hospital for north Dublin, and indeed the country, any further downgrading of Temple Street would not be in anybody's interest.'

Hayes claimed the letter showed that the taoiseach was pressing his minister for health over the allocation and distribution of paediatric services in Dublin on the assumption that the new national children's hospital would be sited at the Mater. However, there was at this time no plan for a single *national* children's hospital, only the long-envisaged rebuilding of Temple Street at the Mater.

I put these issues to Ahern towards the end of a lengthy interview. Of the original plan, to redevelop the Mater and move Temple Street to its campus, he says: 'I was more than happy with that. Of course I was associated with the Mater, but I never lost sleep over where the children's hospital was going. But no, I never spoke to McKinsey or the civil servants doing the review.

'If the idea of a national children's hospital had never come into it, I would have been happier. If I had my way, I'd have favoured one children's hospital on each side of the city. The idea of one location is wrong.'

The southside children's hospitals – Tallaght and Crumlin – dug in. Tallaght said it would not cooperate with the plan for the Mater unless it was changed, and invited Crumlin to discuss creating a new hospital jointly. This proposal went nowhere. Crumlin favoured a single hospital on one site, whereas Tallaght wanted two locations, one northside and the other southside, under the aegis of one hospital.

Crumlin resolved to build a new hospital, either on its site or at a greenfield location. The largest children's hospital in the country withdrew cooperation with the design and planning process for the new facility at the Mater. Public relations advisors were drafted in to promote the hospital's interests in the national media.

It was a time of high emotion. 'I couldn't believe how negative and self-centred some people were,' one of the Crumlin parents campaigning for a new hospital recalls. 'We were dealing with our own very sick children. Yet all one consultant wanted to know was where he could park his car in the new hospital.'

Linda Dillon recalls Mary Harney coming to visit Crumlin around this time. Hospital management had made sure the corridors of the hospital were painted before she arrived, leaving Dillon to wonder: 'Why in God's name would anyone not use the opportunity of a minister's visit to show her the reality?' Still, she managed to divert the minister briefly from the official tour to point out the dowdy cabins where her daughter's high-tech stem-cell treatment had been stored.

Before the minister's tour, Dillon had asked her daughter if there was something she wanted her to tell Harney. Alice, who was seriously ill at the time, replied, 'Just tell her to go and do it.'

The minister received the message and took to repeating it regularly. Alice, sadly, would never get to see the new hospital; she died in July 2006, five years into her treatment for cancer. 'I never really believed we could get away with it,' her mother says. 'She got a few good years. Two years in school. Sleepovers and swimming trips. We were the lucky ones.'

The strength of opposition to the Mater proposal was extraordinary, even by the usual standards of the Irish health service. In the words of an *Irish Times* editorial: 'The rows have revealed the reality that, despite the establishment of a monolithic HSE to run all services and the availability of previously undreamed of resources, the traditional faultlines of Irish healthcare – the medical and local politics, the institutional rivalries, the turf wars, the disagreements over philosophies of care and the involvement of religion – have never gone away.'

That newspaper's columnist Mary Raftery was almost a lone voice urging the government to stand firm: 'The idea that a privately owned hospital such as Crumlin can go off on its own and set up in complete opposition to what is overwhelmingly agreed to be in the best interests of children – namely to have only one tertiary children's hospital in the country – is simply unacceptable.'

For the HSE, Karl Anderson ran workshops on the project for

staff from the different hospitals in its boardroom. At the Temple Street briefing, there was 'applause and palpable excitement'. And then at the Crumlin group, there was silence. 'That spoke volumes.'

Questions were raised about the ownership of the Mater site, but the issue was covered in the task group report. The site for the hospital would be ceded to the state unencumbered and at no cost, and land for a maternity hospital would also be provided.

Ultimately, the opposition to the project came to nothing. Despite all the noise, the Mater plan was the only clear proposal on the table. Its opponents were deeply divided, and unable to come up with an agreed alternative (at one point, there were calls to build the hospital in the Phoenix Park). Proposals from private developers attracted widespread suspicion. Opposition parties, though quick to allege Bertie Ahern's involvement, declined to back an alternative to the Mater. Patient groups, even those linked to Crumlin, lobbied for the hospital to be built as quickly as possible. The public grew impatient for progress to be made.

In January 2007, Apple unveiled the iPhone to the world. That same month, the government formally decided to build a new children's hospital at the Mater. Ministers promised it would be ready by 2011.

Crumlin continued to call for an independent review and Tallaght for a hospital built across two sites, but there was now an inevitability about the government's plans. Even if the dream of a national children's hospital had been poisoned by acrimony and disagreement, it seemed that nothing could stop it from going ahead.

9

Totemic Architecture and the Crash

'The doubts were seeded in my head at an early stage. The Mater site wasn't fit for purpose.'

Philip Lynch, chairman of the National Paediatric Hospital Development Board, which had been tasked with building the children's hospital at the Mater

'Who here has built a hospital?'

Businessman John Gallagher's question to members of the development board he was appointed to chair in October 2010. No one replied.

The sound of shouting could be heard across the floor of the Department of Health. Bemused civil servants stopped work and strained to listen. Behind the minister's door, a good old-fashioned row was gathering force.

It was early October 2010, and Mary Harney had just ushered into her office the man she had appointed to lead the government's flagship project to build a new national children's hospital. Across from her sat Philip Lynch, one of the country's most prominent businessmen. A man more used to calling the shots than being summoned to a meeting at short notice.

So much had changed in Ireland since Lynch took on the job of chairman of the National Paediatric Hospital Development Board more than three years earlier. With the economy going into freefall, little of it was good. Few were spared the fallout from this national calamity and both Harney and Lynch, in their separate ways, were feeling the pressure. And now, between them, the fate of the government's prestige building project hung in the balance.

To great fanfare, the go-ahead for the new hospital at the Mater had been given in 2007. Very soon, though, it was clear that the timing was terrible. Just as government green-lit the project, a subprime mortgage crisis was kicking off in the US. A full-blown global financial crisis followed soon after. Ireland's Celtic Tiger economy, more extended than most, crashed. A property bubble led to the collapse of the banking system, eventually forcing the country to seek a bailout from the European Union and the International Monetary Fund in 2010. Unemployment tripled, public debt soared and emigration grew to levels not seen since the 1980s. The public mood grew angrier as the government struggled to balance the books.

The crisis impacted heavily on the health service. Almost €3 billion was cut from health spending; staff numbers in the HSE were reduced by 12,000. Waiting list and hospital trolley numbers soared. In Crumlin, almost 1,000 operations were cancelled in the first half of 2009. The state's biggest children's hospital was forced to postpone two vitally needed heart operations every week.

Building the new children's hospital remained official policy, though for now no one in government was in any hurry to start spending serious money on its construction. Brendan Drumm knew that the hospital was likely to swallow most of the HSE's capital budget for years to come. But once his term as head of the HSE was up in 2010, there was no guarantee that the next person running the health service would show as much interest as he had.

To ensure that the project survived his departure, he had already in 2006 suggested the creation of an independent board, appointed by government, to build and then run the hospital. The search for a potential chairperson to propose to the minister took several months before Drumm approached Philip Lynch. The Corkman had made his name by rescuing the Irish Agricultural Wholesale Society (IAWS), a food business with roots in the cooperative movement. That struck a chord with Drumm, arising from his father's work with co-ops in the northwest.

After IAWS, Lynch had moved on to One51, which became the go-to investment firm of the Celtic Tiger years but tanked later as the economic bubble fully burst. Drumm remembers inviting the businessman to meet Harney for the first time: 'He had this huge chauffeur-driven Lexus car, a big long thing. I remember her laughing, saying, "Why don't ministers get one of these?"'

Lynch recalls telling his wife about the offer to become chairman of the hospital development board. 'She said, "You must be mad.

What are you doing that for? Do you not have enough to do?" I told her that I wanted to put something back, to make a difference.'

Harney duly appointed Lynch chairman in March 2007, charged with delivering the new facility on a site adjacent to the Mater adult hospital. The 12-person board was formally established two months later.

The three children's hospitals were allotted a seat each on the development board. Doctors from Temple Street and Tallaght took up theirs. Crumlin boycotted the new body. Other appointees included Crumlin parent Linda Dillon, a brace of HSE officials and two prominent figures – nurse-turned-magazine publisher Norah Casey and property developer and entrepreneur Harry Crosbie.

'I was really excited to be part of the biggest building project in the Irish state, and for such a great cause,' Casey recalls. 'We'd been given a fait accompli, but we still all felt the Mater was absolutely the right site. We had reviewed the site ourselves and saw where the footprint would be. At that stage, everyone was on board. This was the right place.'

The group's first challenges were banal, practical ones. There was no infrastructure and funding was hard to access. Without premises or staff, even a chief executive, the board met in Casey's or Lynch's offices. The board's first annual report was designed and printed by Casey's company, because no public funding was available. At one point, it couldn't place job advertisements in the newspapers because there were no funds in the bank to pay for them.

Preparatory work for the hospital got underway. In March 2007, UK consultants RKW (Rawlinson Kelly & Whittlestone) were engaged to draw up a planning framework for the project.

In a series of subsequent reports from RKW, the hospital was given outline shape – single en-suite rooms for all patients with parent accommodation, a cap of about 400 beds and the creation of urgent-care centres in the greater Dublin area to complement the main children's hospital. The first should be in Tallaght, the consultants recommended, and the second in Blanchardstown. A third, possibly in Loughlinstown, to the south of Dublin, was also suggested. The project had started growing.

Crumlin's boycott of the development board made it hard to plan for the transfer of services. 'It was difficult to know what they wanted, but they definitely didn't want the Mater,' according to Casey. 'Mostly they wanted ownership of the project. At times it appeared they wanted the new hospital developed on their site or James's, but later they wanted a greenfield site. It was definitely a case of "anywhere but the Mater".'

Harney assured Crumlin she would walk away from the Mater if RKW found there wasn't enough space there for a children's hospital. The consultants didn't deal with this issue in detail because a wider review of maternity services was ongoing at the time, but their report mentioned that there *was* sufficient space available for a future maternity hospital at the Mater.

'A building of the requisite scale can be accommodated on the site in line with urban developments elsewhere on the assumption that a cleared site will be available and within an overall site development capacity of 140,000 square metres,' the report also stated. 'There are many examples of children's hospitals in buildings of comparable density and height to that which is likely to result from a development on the Mater site.'

That might be the case in other cities, but it hardly took account of Dublin's low-rise heritage. An opportunity was missed here to try to increase the footprint of the Mater site so that a lower building could be designed.

As the economic outlook worsened, state coffers emptied and the long finger became an active instrument of government policy. The project ran into problems. In February 2008, Lynch told Brendan Drumm in a letter that delays in transferring ownership of the site from the nuns were placing board members in a 'very difficult and embarrassing position'.

Although Lynch was under 'no illusions' about how the public system worked compared to the private sector, 'nothing could have prepared me for what is the current debacle in which we find ourselves', he told Drumm. 'There is huge apathy and antipathy towards this project and there are many very public detractors. This is all the more reason why one would expect the HSE and its executives would give us every assistance, support and encouragement in our mammoth task.'

He was 'mystified' how these matters could be 'so badly managed and handled. If such basic issues cannot be managed in the initial stages of the process, how can we have confidence in relation to issues management when we get into the middle of an €800 million to €1 billion project?'

In March 2009, former nurse and deputy chief executive of St James's Hospital, Eilish Hardiman, was appointed the first chief executive of the development board. Together, staff and board members started planning in detail the new hospital that would arise in Dublin's city centre.

There was a further breakthrough that year when Crumlin agreed to take up its seat on the development board. 'People went overboard to get Crumlin back to the table,' says one manager familiar with the project at this time. 'Their every whim was catered for.'

There was a downside to this willingness to facilitate Crumlin, the manager claims. As a result, 'the hospital grew and grew', as more and better facilities were promised to the doctors who would work in it.

Casey, though, insists planning was conducted 'in a robust way. Costs were going to be nailed down so that the project didn't run over. Harry [Crosbie] and I were used to the language of procurement and how to avoid pitfalls in the contracts, so there was no wriggle room for suppliers to start increasing costs.'

Despite this progress, funding worries increased. With the economy in collapse, where was the money to come from? Already, the cost of the hospital had increased from an initial estimate of €500 million, to €650 million. Philanthropy was supposed to magic up €110 million of this but nothing had yet been raised, and prospects were poor, given the downturn and criticism from those who favoured a different location for the hospital. Equipping the new facility with computers would cost €100 million, it was estimated, but this was not budgeted for.

Architects were appointed and a planning application prepared for the hospital, but still opposition persisted. 'The most difficult part of those first few years was the disgruntlement and constant criticism of the site from Crumlin and other detractors,' Casey recalls.

In 2009, then taoiseach Brian Cowen promised the hospital

would open by the end of 2014. In just two years, the timeline for the project had slipped by three years.

As preparations for the new hospital inched forward and the country's economic fortunes continued to stagnate, renowned heart surgeon Maurice Neligan, an early supporter of the Mater proposal, did a prominent volte-face. Writing in his weekly *Irish Times* column in July 2010, Neligan said his original position had been wrong.

'Neither the Mater nor the joint children's hospitals may be best served by this proposed development on a geographically constrained site,' he wrote. Ireland's economic crash should prompt a rethink: 'Given our present economic circumstances, this project is not about totemic architecture, however excellent. It is about sick children and their families.'

Calling instead for the renovation of Crumlin, he argued that 'a much more modest investment on its current site and agreed staffing levels would hold the fort until the sun shines again'.

Without any elaboration, Neligan claimed that the original recommendation for colocating the children's hospital with an adult teaching hospital was 'dubious'. 'It is not specified why this should be the case,' he wrote – an assertion that ignored the lengthy reasoning on this point in the McKinsey report.

'Crucial decisions were made on limited and selective criteria and without honest debate among those most qualified at home to give advice, and driven by concerns far beyond the welfare of the children,' the surgeon continued. When the hospital was eventually built, he argued, this should happen on 'a greenfield site, spacious and easy of access'.

Neligan had carried out Ireland's first heart transplant and was revered by colleagues and patients alike. In retirement, his regular newspaper musings had a loyal following. It might just have been the view of one person, but his change of heart was devastating for the Mater cause. (Neligan died suddenly in October 2010, just three months after this column was published.)

Lynch too was starting to have second thoughts. 'The doubts were seeded in my head at an early stage,' he says. 'The Mater site wasn't fit for purpose. If this was going to make any sense, the children's hospital had to be beside a maternity hospital.'

The new hospital was being shoehorned into an already busy site, he felt, where there were problems with parking, overshadowing of local houses and fitting in with plans for an underground metro stop. Further, he noted, there was 'no appetite' in the three existing children's hospitals for amalgamation. And, at least in his opinion, no space at the Mater for a maternity hospital.

Meetings of the development board grew increasingly fractious. 'He didn't understand the public sector base to the project,' says one member of the board of its chairman. 'He had an antipathy to civil servants. There was a feeling of "we know how to do this but you don't". But we were trying to build a hospital and, at that stage, we didn't even own the site.'

Lynch denies being frustrated at the speed at which the project was moving. As a former chairman of An Post, he was well familiar with the public sector, he points out, and appreciated it moved at a different pace. Behind the scenes, he started investigating other options.

Four years after he had first proposed developing the children's hospital on land near Tallaght, southwest of the city, solicitor-turned-developer Noel Smyth wrote a letter to *The Irish Times* repeating the offer of a private build. He claimed he could deliver this for €150 million less than it would cost at the Mater.

Lynch contacted Smyth after reading the letter. He also met representatives from Crumlin hospital, and then he formulated a plan to move the entire project to Smyth's land. 'Here was 30 acres of land, well situated, free of charge. It was an ideal site, and it would have accommodated the maternity hospital too. It was a good idea,' he tells me in a telephone interview.

By now Jonathan Irwin, former bloodstock agent and founder of Jack and Jill Children's Foundation, a well-regarded charity providing respite care for very sick children, had joined the opposition to the Mater plan. 'Many of our families are greatly distressed at the thought of trying to find the Mater and struggling through the maze of one-way streets to get there in an emergency,' the Eton-educated Irwin suggested. He too wanted the project to be relocated to the periphery of Dublin, where families from outside the capital could access it easily via the M50 ring road.

Smyth's plan again gained considerable traction in the media, though he had never built a hospital before. A television station sent out reporters to drive from various parts of the country to Tallaght, St James's and the Mater; from each location, journey times to his site in Tallaght were lowest. Straw polls conducted on radio phone-in shows suggested overwhelming opposition to the Mater.

'The development board lost the public relations battle on this for years and years,' says Jonathan Hourihane, a paediatrician who was later appointed a member of the development board.

'The board's PR was all reactive,' he says, while doctors opposed to the project used their 'moral leverage' with families to promote 'utopian views' of the planned hospital.

Brendan Drumm was dismissive of Smyth's offer at the time, and remains so today. 'The "not for profit" basis of the offer was interpreted by the public as a gift to the state. As with all free gifts, the devil was in the detail. Unlike traditional voluntary hospitals, this hospital would have operated like a private hospital, with a bill issued to the HSE for each patient treated.

'Such a proposal could never be accepted by anybody responsible for taxpayers' money. It would essentially be a monopoly, in a position to demand whatever fees it wished. This would have been an open chequebook arrangement.'

But why not just accept the offer of land and let the state take it from there? 'A standalone site was never going to be acceptable following the recommendations of the different reports. In any case, the state was getting the land free already, irrespective of which public hospital it went to.'

Lynch's thoughts of moving the project to a greenfield site provoked a furious row at the development board. He says individual board members 'aligned to Harney' complained to the minister about his change of heart.

That resulted in Lynch being summoned at short notice to the meeting with the minister in her office in October 2010.

Harney didn't mince her words, as he recalls: 'Your remit is to put this on the Mater. If you won't do this, I want your resignation,' she said.

'I won't give it,' Lynch replied. 'You'll have to fire me first.'

The minster did just that.

Harney doesn't dispute Lynch's version of what happened at the meeting. Asked if she did fire Lynch, she replies, 'I probably did. If he says I did, then I did. By going out in public as chairman of the board saying he wasn't for the project, he was undermining it.'

In a brief statement issued after the meeting, her department announced the 'resignation' of Lynch. Harney is quoted as thanking him for his 'time and dedication for bringing this project to where it is today'.

Lynch released his own press statement after his departure, citing 'significant and fundamental differences' with Harney on key issues. The businessman also wrote a resignation letter highlighting a substantial gap in funding for the project, planning and design challenges at the Mater site, and certain governance issues.

The project had little money and little public support, and now it had no leader.

A brief postscript to Lynch's involvement with the hospital occurred six months after he was sacked. In March 2011, he returned to the headlines, alleging political interference in the decision to put the children's hospital at the Mater.

'It was a political decision, a northside job, I've no doubt in the world about it,' he declared during a radio interview. Bertie Ahern had promised the Sisters of Mercy – the order running the Mater – that they would 'get their hospital', he claimed.

The nuns and Ahern denied the allegation, for which Lynch offered no evidence. The claim ignores the fact that Ahern would have required support from Harney and Drumm to get his way. As mentioned, both deny that there was anything untoward about the process.

'You don't have to admire either person to acknowledge that there is no way they would be party to placing Ahern's constituency imperatives ahead of the health of the nation's children,' Michael Clifford commented at the time in the *Irish Examiner*. 'Harney, it is worth recalling, was the one who put the kibosh in Ahern's ultimate pet project, the Bertie Bowl.'

The 'northside job' allegation would haunt the project for years, despite a lack of evidence. 'I tackled everybody about that in the early days,' Norah Casey says of the claim that Ahern had influenced the process. 'He didn't [have any involvement]. It had nothing to do with him.'

Leo Varadkar, a young TD in west Dublin, joined the cabinet in March as minister for transport, tourism and sport. Varadkar was a medical doctor who had trained in Crumlin and worked in its emergency department for a time. His father was a GP, and his sister a paediatrician.

He says he followed the children's hospital story from the time the McKinsey report was published. 'When I was a councillor, I was of the view that the best thing to do was to go for a greenfield site and new build,' he tells me in an interview conducted in late 2025, a year after his retirement from politics. Despite his earlier views, and his Fine Gael background, he says he 'always thought this stuff about Bertie pulling strings was rubbish'.

He adds: 'There can be unconscious bias sometimes – like when the boundary commission redraws the boundaries, they do know where the party leaders live and rarely carve up their constituencies. But I don't think he actually would have interfered, to be honest, and certainly not directly.'

When I ask Philip Lynch if he had any evidence to support the allegation, he replies, 'No, but I believed it.'

Lynch bowed out of the children's hospital story at this point. Some years later, in 2022, he became the first person in Ireland found to have engaged in insider trading. A Central Bank panel sanctioned him for using inside information to acquire 200,000 shares in a drinks company for his retirement fund. He was publicly cautioned, fined €75,000 and disqualified from being involved in a financial services company for five years.

The insider trading dated back to 2008, when Lynch was a non-executive director of drinks group C&C. At the time, he was also serving as chairman of the National Paediatric Hospital Development Board. Asked if this trading activity had impacted on his involvement with the hospital project, he says his work for the development board was always unaffected.

Harney immediately turned to another businessman on the development board to steady the ship. In contrast to his predecessor as chairman, John Gallagher was low-profile, cautious and analytical. A serial entrepreneur, his first big money was earned in the waste industry and from selling alarms. With his wife Bernie, a member of the Doyle hotel family, he made a fortune from the sale of Dublin hotels at the peak of the market, before the property crash. Gallagher had plenty of experience of construction and big property deals.

Chairing his first meeting of the board, he asked, 'Who here has built a hospital?'

No one replied.

'Anyone here ever build a house?' he then asked.

Again, silence.

A change in the external environment was looming, which would have a big impact on oversight of the project in the Department of Health. The general election, held in February 2011, was effectively a referendum on the Fianna Fáil/Green coalition's handling of the financial crisis. The result was never in doubt; Fianna Fáil saw its first-preference votes halved while Fine Gael and Labour swept to power with a combined 58-seat majority.

Harney, who had resigned as minister for health a month earlier, did not contest the general election. A mould-breaking early political career ultimately foundered on the many crises thrown up by the health service and Ireland's economic collapse. She largely disappeared from public life thereafter.

Drumm, meanwhile, had returned to academia and clinical practice in 2010 after the end of his bruising five-year term as HSE chief executive. The two original supporters of the plan for a single children's hospital were no longer leading the health service.

James Reilly, a businessman, GP and former president of the

Irish Medical Organisation, was appointed minister for health in March 2011. The craggy-faced, bearded Reilly had been a combative health spokesman in opposition. If he had limited political experience, he had no experience of political office. 'Clever, polite and sometimes narky,' a cabinet colleague says of him: 'He had that doctor thing of being sure of his opinions.'

In opposition, Reilly and his party had been unenthusiastic about the Mater plan, though it wasn't clear what new approach they favoured. Before the election, he and Fine Gael leader Enda Kenny had met Eilish Hardiman and asked about the cost of building the hospital off the M50. Gallagher had also met Reilly and came away with the impression that the project could well be relocated if Fine Gael got into power.

As minister, Reilly was inheriting a project that was closely associated with the *ancien régime* – Harney certainly and, whether he wanted it or not, Ahern. Inevitably, there was speculation that the new minister would seek to revise the existing plan, perhaps by changing the location.

'It wasn't my ambition before I became minister to build the new children's hospital,' Reilly tells me. 'And it wasn't my brainchild either, but I was very happy to progress it. And, as a northsider, I would have been delighted for it to be at the Mater.'

Now Fine Gael *was* in power, along with Labour. Gallagher fretted about continuing in a post that was intimately linked to the Mater location, when the hospital might end up somewhere else. Millions had been spent there in preparation for the children's hospital, and the development board was locked into expensive contracts on the Mater site. Who would end up carrying the can if the location was changed but the chairman of the development board remained in place? He decided to seek specific assurances from the new minister before carrying on in the job.

Gallagher wrote to Reilly congratulating him on his appointment and revealing that he had conducted his own review of the project. 'I asked myself, if it was my own money, would I still do the project in its current form?' he told the minister in the March 2011 letter.

The businessman had brought in experts in architecture, property, law and finance to run the rule over the Mater site. They reviewed the project positively: subject to final costings, the project had 'very strong merit' and could be substantially completed in a single term of government.

However, he told the minister, the project as then structured was 'unworkable'. External contractors and consultants were not being properly managed, he claimed, because the executive team was unable to handle the large numbers of 'change orders' – written instructions about changes to a job already in progress, and the costs involved – generated.

Gallagher's warning about the difficulty of managing contract changes and external contractors proved prophetic, as the issue would become a recurring problem when construction of the hospital got underway.

He also wanted structural changes to ensure that construction happened promptly and came in on budget. For a start, he felt, an independent board was needed for a project of this size. Either the HSE should take over the running of the project or funding should be managed by experts in the National Development Finance

Agency (NDFA). He estimated the cost of building the hospital at a minimum €615 million.

The NDFA had a prominent role in overseeing many state construction projects, it was true, but it tended to use the public private partnership (PPP) model, where a private company financed and built the piece of infrastructure. While this had worked well in providing schools and motorways, the children's hospital was regarded by the Department of Health as too complex for a PPP.

'It would have been a massive financing risk given the length of build. The market would have charged a lot of money to finance it. And the risk premium would be too high,' according to an informed source. The level of maintenance required for a children's hospital over time was also seen as too unpredictable for such an arrangement.

Gallagher had a crucial final ask now that work was at a 'critical juncture': he wanted the 'open and full' support of the minister and the government. A failure to endorse the clinical case for the Mater would 'fatally compromise' the project and increase the cost of delivery, he warned.

'Significant structural changes' were needed 'within a short time period,' he warned. Otherwise, 'I would find it difficult to continue in the role.'

Meeting Reilly in a hotel near his north Dublin home in June 2026, I ask him why he didn't give Gallagher the support he was looking for. 'Look at the date [9 March 2011],' he replies. '[I was] ... only in the gate after the election of 25 February. [It was] far too early to be making those type of undertakings '

Gallagher followed up his letter with a request for a meeting.

He was kept waiting for a time before being admitted to the minister's office for the appointment. Explaining that his remit extended solely to building a hospital at the Mater, he delivered an ultimatum: the minister needed to commit to the Mater plan, or he (Gallagher) would resign. And he would do this at six o'clock that evening.

Through his secretary, the minister asked Gallagher not to resign. But he gave no commitment to sticking with the Mater. Gallagher resigned. The development board had lost its second chairman in six months. To fill the gap, Harry Crosbie was elected interim chairman.

Two weeks later, in April 2011, Reilly announced an independent review of the project, saying he wanted a clear estimate of the costs involved. Never mind that three previous reviews had been conducted – McKinsey, the task group of civil servants and RKW consultants – all reaching broadly similar conclusions. To avoid accusations of bias, international experts were appointed to lead this latest review. A UK architect was engaged to do an initial analysis, which was followed by a clinical assessment by the chief executives of hospitals in Boston and Denver in the US, and Brisbane in Australia.

'I insisted on one key parameter: the main purpose of this hospital was to ensure we could treat as many children with rare conditions in the country, so they wouldn't have to go abroad,' Reilly says. 'We needed the maximum number of tertiary specialists in rare conditions working there.'

The same thinking had underpinned Reilly's initiative in developing an all-Ireland paediatric cardiac service, a successful initiative that has saved many children the arduous trip to England for surgery.

The group he appointed drafted a report stating that 'the ideal location would be located on green space' and be trilocated with adult and maternity hospitals. It mentioned that St James's, as a high level adult teaching hospital, also met the colocation criteria, even if it presented 'similar if not more constraints' to those identified at the Mater.

The reference to an ideal site was removed from the final report by the chairman of the review panel, who reasoned that it would lead to claims that there was indeed such a place. Ultimately, and ironically given Gallagher's premature departure, the report endorsed the Mater site. Published in July 2011, the review concluded that it would be no cheaper to build the hospital on a greenfield site, given that millions had already been spent on planning the hospital on the Mater campus. Changing location, it was said, would delay the project by another eight years.

The final report noted that 'no perfect site' was available, and suggested that the traffic and access issues raised at the Mater could be 'mitigated' even if a planned metro line underneath never went ahead. Colocating the hospital with an adult facility and a maternity hospital was 'essential to the development of an excellent paediatric service'.

Four separate reviews had now affirmed the principle of colocating the children's hospital with an adult hospital and three of them had explicitly given the Mater the thumbs-up for the project. More time had been lost; the expected completion date had slipped another year, to 2015.

10

'The political system blew a gasket'

'... if there is going to be a building towering over a city, much better that it's a children's hospital than a rugby stadium.'

Norah Casey, member of the development board, tasked with building the children's hospital at the Mater, 2007–12

'... with respect to Dorset Street, it is not the Champs-Élysées.'

An 'incandescent' Senator John Crown, criticising An Bord Pleanála's refusal of planning permission for the Mater site, and its observation that the proposed building would overlook Dorset Street

On the morning of 15 September 2011, residents of Dublin woke up to the impression that a giant ocean liner had docked in the middle of their city.

There it stood in a photograph in that morning's newspapers, multiple lines of cabins visible above a massive hull, towering behind a duck pond and the jumble of small red-brick houses in the inner city, its giant wall of shimmering glass broken by just the occasional splash of yellow. The new arrival was one of the highest structures in Dublin, visible from O'Connell Street, the Phoenix Park and many other parts of the city.

This behemoth wasn't actually an ocean liner, but a photomontage of the proposed new children's hospital at the Mater. What looked like tiny cabins in the picture were bedrooms, and the yellow flecks were balconies.

The scheme, designed by architects O'Connell Mahon, proposed an eight-storey rectangular block topped by an oval-shaped element that would also be eight storeys high. Overall the building would be 74 metres tall – over 14 metres higher than Liberty Hall.

'This oval-shaped structure looks for all the world like a football stadium, and bears a remarkable resemblance to the Aviva Stadium at Lansdowne Road,' local residents said in their submission to An Bord Pleanála. 'To even consider this proposed development on a site such as the Mater beggars belief,' they added, citing its elevated position, the proximity of protected structures such as the Francis Johnston-designed St George's Church and the surrounding residential environment.

The various photomontages of the scheme, prepared for an environmental impact statement as part of the planning application, raised eyebrows. The project had been allowed to bypass the local authority stage for planning applications because it was deemed strategic infrastructure. These photomontages were Dubliners' first look at the proposed building.

'It was a massive project,' Dr Mary Kelly, who was chairwoman of An Bord Pleanála at the time, tells me. 'I remember seeing the scale model of the building in the hallway of our offices, saying, "Crikey, that's huge", and realising what a massive decision it would be.'

Over at the Custom House, Department of Environment planning official John Martin saw the same images and said to himself: 'That project's in trouble.'

I too recall seeing the photomontages in the newspaper that morning and thinking, *How is this ever going to get through planning?*

An Taisce, in its submission to the planning board, warned that the design was 'seriously over-scaled [and] damaging to the setting and integrity of protected structures' and residential streets. 'The site is inherently unsuitable for a new National Children's Hospital because of its constricted nature,' the conservation body said.

If the photomontages didn't set alarm bells ringing more widely, it may have been because many still cleaved to the belief that the Mater plan was a done deal – the 'northside job' referred to by Philip Lynch. After all, it was said, wasn't the planning application being fast-tracked with An Bord Pleanála under the relatively new strategic infrastructure legislation?

The latest review of the project by overseas experts had delayed progress, but once Reilly gave a fresh go-ahead in July 2011, the planning application for the Mater site had been lodged immediately.

Far from being assuaged by the findings of the independent review, opposition to the Mater had continued to simmer. Now, with the proposed design of the building looking so misplaced, it boiled up again. 'The incredible hulk' was the name given it by *Irish Times* environment editor Frank McDonald. 'It is hard not to conclude that the Mater must be the wrong site, especially given its sensitive location in Dublin's northside Georgian core,' he argued. 'Just because €31 million has already been racked up should not mean that it cannot be cancelled.'

Building the hospital at St James's instead would allow for lateral expansion, because its site was four times the size of the Mater's, McDonald reasoned. In contrast, 'building upwards' would be the only option at the Mater should further expansion be required. 'An Bord Pleanála would be doing the old, the sick and the disabled – not to mention taxpayers – a big favour by refusing permission,' he concluded.

An Bord Pleanála decided to hold an oral hearing – a public meeting to discuss the project – before one of its inspectors. When this got underway in October, the enormous scale of the project dominated proceedings.

With the design likened to a multi-deck cruise ship sitting on top of a nine-storey building, it was clear the hospital would be visible across the city. Its impact would be altogether different from that of a more slender tower.

Still, few expected An Bord Pleanála to refuse permission for such a flagship project, located in a recent taoiseach's constituency and backed by the line minister and head of the health service. 'It would not be surprising if the board eventually gives its approval for the scheme; after all, it represents the realisation of Government policy, which the board would be loathe to ignore,' was McDonald's prediction in the first week of the three-week hearing.

The oral hearing completed, An Bord Pleanála proceeded to deliberate, its decision anxiously awaited by both supporters and opponents of the Mater scheme. However, the planning body had its own problems.

By the end of 2011, it had been reduced to just four members, none of them an architect, and there was no indication when further appointments would be made.

Minister for environment Phil Hogan had declined to reappoint two architects and one planner when their terms of office had ended that December. This was despite An Bord Pleanála requesting a two-year extension.

The minister pointed out that the appointments were his prerogative and that some of the members who were not reappointed had served multiple terms.

'I'd love you to try and get to the bottom of what happened in An Bord Pleanála,' Bertie Ahern tells me when I interview him for this book. His suggestion seems to be that this in some way influenced the outcome of the hospital's planning application.

'We were left short of members on the board for ages, despite making requests for appointments to be made,' Mary Kelly, its then chairwoman, explains when I ask her. 'It wasn't unusual for a state board to experience this, even if it was serious for a busy planning body like ours. Neither was it unusual to have a split decision.'

Whatever the reasons for the gaps left on the board, the Mater planning application was clearly going to be affected. A decision on the state's biggest construction project would be made late, by a depleted board.

In February 2012, seven months after the planning application was submitted, An Bord Pleanála made public its decision, reached by a three to one majority. Planning permission was refused on grounds of the scale and impact on the environment.

The proposed hospital would result in a 'dominant, visually incongruous structure' with 'a profound negative impact' on the city skyline and would 'seriously detract' from the character of local streetscapes, it ruled. The project amounted to 'overdevelopment of the Mater campus' and was found to be contrary to the proper planning and sustainable development of the area.

The decision came as a shock to politicians and the development board alike. 'The political system blew a gasket,' a source familiar with the planning system recalls. 'It was regarded as outrageous that An Bord Pleanála would have the cheek to refuse a project of such national significance.'

Tony O'Brien remembers the decision well, having taken on responsibility for hospitals policy in the Department of Health on the same day that the planners made their announcement. 'There was shock and anger – shock from the civil servants and anger from the politicians. The politicians felt that they'd been given high levels of assurance by the civil servants [in the Department of Health] that the planning application wouldn't be a problem, that there had been contact and preplanning discussions with An Bord Pleanála and so on. They were heading into that week fully confident they could get planning approval.

'James Reilly, less than a year into the job, was annoyed. He had had some misgivings about the Eccles Street site [the Mater campus] but had been given such a high degree of assurance that he felt he shouldn't interfere with it. If he had questioned the project without good reason, he would just have been delaying it.'

Publicly, Taoiseach Enda Kenny expressed disappointment but promised the government would still build the hospital within its lifetime. An independent review was promised to decide what would happen next.

'That's when it all fell asunder,' Norah Casey recalls. The development board felt 'blindsided' by the planners' decision, she says, but still believed it could deliver on the Mater site: 'The whole point in working with An Bord Pleanála on huge capital infrastructure projects is that there are no surprises on either side. They're supposed to be guiding and steering. Yet we were constantly asking for an update when the decision was delayed.'

Earlier in her career, Casey had worked as a nurse in London, in big hospitals reaching skywards in crowded downtown locations. She had visited the much-lauded Starship children's hospital in Auckland while serving on the development board in order to get ideas about what could be done in Ireland. The Starship is the biggest children's hospital in New Zealand and a dominant structure in its largest city, she points out: 'That's as it should be, because it's a hospital that is catering for the whole of New Zealand and the future.'

Casey argues that hospitals are better designed 'up and down' (using lifts) rather than being spread out as it's easier and more efficient for staff to get around. 'Personally, I felt that if there was going to be a building towering over a city, much better that it's a children's hospital than a rugby stadium,' she says, in reference to the then recently constructed Aviva Stadium.

But another board member, who declined to be named, feels that the new hospital was 'over-specced' even at this early stage. The design was heading 'out of control' with 'way too much leeway' given to clinical and other demands, he says. This might explain why the proposed building was so large, at 16 storeys.

Bertie Ahern, the politician most associated with the Mater, was by now four years into his political retirement but still deeply mired in controversy. For years, the Mahon tribunal had been scrutinising his personal finances, in particular large, unexplained cash lodgements to his account when he was minister for finance in the 1990s. Its final report, published in March 2012, weeks after the planning refusal for the hospital, rejected much of the explanation he gave about this as untrue.

'I was disappointed with the An Bord Pleanála decision, and annoyed,' Ahern says. 'There was no argument on transport and colocation with a general hospital. Consultants had sorted out the ethos. The design team's work was well advanced, and three reviews [four, in fact] had been carried out into the site.

'The grounds for turning down the Mater were totally spurious; that if you were walking up O'Connell Street, you'd see this building rising up behind the Ambassador cinema. What a load of bull. What would be affected? There's high-rise buildings all over now.'

Independent senator and oncologist Professor John Crown made a similar point at the time planning permission was refused. The proposed site at the Mater was bordered on one side by a prison and on the other by two hospitals, he pointed out. It overlooked Dorset Street, and 'with respect to Dorset Street it is not the Champs-Élysées'.

Fourteen years on from her planning board's decision, Mary Kelly has no regrets. 'The building was too big for its location. From O'Connell Bridge, it would have towered over O'Connell Street, and there were also traffic and parking issues. We were very conscious of the importance of the decision, the absolute need for a new children's hospital, but when it was assessed on objective planning grounds it did not stand up.'

Asked about the independence of the process, she says, 'I was never approached by anyone seeking to influence the decision and there was no political interference. I would have cried foul if there had been.'

In March, just weeks after the Mater decision, Phil Hogan filled the vacant seats on An Bord Pleanála. One of his appointees was an architect.

While researching this book, I contacted An Coimisiún Pleanála, the successor planning body to An Bord Pleanála since 2025, seeking access to the environmental impact study (EIS) for the Mater project.

This document would contain the damaging photomontages showing the proposed hospital building dominating the skyline in central Dublin, which were probably key to the project being rejected. I also asked for the minutes of the four board meetings at which the case was considered in February 2012. The decision was a split one, and I wanted to know why.

The public has a right of access to such documents, even if, because of the amount of time elapsed, they are held in storage rather than being readable online.

However, these documents, relating to one of the biggest construction projects ever planned in the state, are not available. An official replied saying they no longer had a copy of the EIS, apart from a short non-technical summary, and did not have any records of meetings for cases dating from before 2014. Efforts by staff to get copies of the photomontages from other sources came to nothing.

As a result, I was unable to review the original images in the EIS, the ones that had caused such a fuss before the board made its decision on the planning application at the Mater. The lack of board minutes meant there was no public record of the internal discussions that took place, or why the outcome was a split vote.

11

'The most dispiriting project'

'Peacock today, feather-duster tomorrow!'

The warning businessman Frank Dolphin received from his sister upon being appointed chairman of the HSE in July 2010

'It was the best process for the resources, capability and time we had.'

Dolphin, on the work of the review group he chaired on the selection of a new site for the children's hospital

Frank Dolphin was lecturing a group of students on organisational psychology one day, emphasising the importance of leadership, when one asked, 'If it's so important to be a leader, then why are you talking about it rather than actually becoming one?'

Dolphin had no answer. But he did have a 'light-bulb moment', realising it was time to try something new, to leave his pensionable job and take a risk. From the front room of his house in Waterford, he started a call-centre business, remortgaging it to fund further growth. It was to be the start of a successful career in business process outsourcing in Europe and the US, built on call centres and other firms employing thousands of staff.

Long before his foray into business he had worked as a clinical psychologist in Temple Street. Around 2007, at the height of his entrepreneurial career, the hospital came calling, asking him to serve on its board. Within a year, he was appointed chair.

Originally from Birr, County Offaly, and living well outside Dublin, Dolphin was something of an outsider to medical politics in the capital, while being intimately familiar with Temple Street's challenges. He tried to mend fences between the children's hospitals by bringing their boards together for a historic joint meeting in 2008. 'The relationship between the three hospitals was non-existent,' he recalls. 'A lot of the time, consultants in one hospital didn't get on with consultants in the other, and that spilled over into an antipathy between the hospitals at times. Allied to that, the hospitals were competing for resources and funding.'

His efforts came to the attention of Mary Harney, who appointed him chair of the HSE in July 2010. 'Remember: peacock today, feather-duster tomorrow,' his sister warned him at the time.

Her prediction seemed to prove accurate when Dolphin had to step down after little more than a year. Harney had departed politics and James Reilly, the new broom in the Department of Health, was proposing governance reforms that would see the HSE abolished. (Ultimately, it wasn't.)

In the pandemonium that followed the rejection of planning permission for the children's hospital, it fell to the relatively new minister to decide what to do next.

'I was concerned,' Reilly says. 'The project at the Mater was considered to be a dead duck, so we were leaving €36 million behind.'

He says he was infuriated by the reaction from some of those involved in designing the hospital. 'It didn't seem to cost them at all that this money was gone. They seemed to have ignored the planning signals they got during the application, and just persisted. It was a slap in the face for the taxpayer, with so much money spent on the project.'

Reilly set up yet another review group and asked Dolphin to chair it, just four months after he had stepped down from his HSE role.

The businessman was given 56 days – extended on request to 70 – to advise on a way forward. Reilly appointed four doctors to the review group, along with an architect, two planners and a British hospital executive.

'The minister wanted to move things on fast, to move this issue off his desk,' says Dolphin. The group had 'absolutely minimal resources. We were given a disused office to work out of. We had no budget. But that was just the reality of the time'. It was the height of the financial crisis.

'The politicians scurried about looking for a solution to this problem for which they were now accountable,' says Tony O'Brien. 'They set about doing everything they could to move it towards the St James's site.'

'Department of Health officials were utterly shell-shocked by the Mater decision. They did not see it coming,' says John Martin, appointed to the Dolphin group after retiring from his planning role at the Department of the Environment. 'Something like €40 million in public funds had gone down the drain there, so it was very important from their point of view that they didn't get another unexpected planning refusal.'

With his expertise, Martin realised the biggest drawback of the Mater scheme was a lack of expansion space. 'An Bord Pleanála itself was not clear a maternity hospital would fit there. Even when they spread the building out and brought the height down from 16 storeys, that made it very bulky.' His job, and that of the other planner on the group, was to make sure the same mistake was not made again.

Still, both the Mater and the development board were insisting that the planning issues that had emerged during the oral hearing could be resolved. Harry Crosbie, who lived in the inner city and was instrumental in reviving the Docklands area, talked up a revised bid at the Mater, promising to create 'an intimate tree-lined and beautiful collegiate workplace' on the site.

Late in the day, the nuns running the Mater made extra land and buildings available, allowing for the size of the site to be increased by one-third. This, it was claimed, would allow a reduction in the height of the building to ten storeys – still high by the standards of the time. The boards of the Mater, Temple Street and the nearby Rotunda hospital jointly announced that an adjacent piece of land was 'shovel-ready' for a new maternity hospital, to which the Rotunda could move.

Drawing on his experience in the entertainment business, Crosbie, who had developed the Point Theatre (now 3Arena), the Bord Gáis Energy Theatre and Vicar Street, promised to put on a 'spectacular' stadium concert to kick-start fundraising for the project.

But the development board, lacking health or political support, was fighting an increasingly lonely battle. Members were keen to rework their plans but the minister seemed unenthusiastic.

'We were back to another review of the location, instead of standing up to An Bord Pleanála and saying, "work with the team, let's make this happen"', Casey says.

Publicly, Reilly insisted that 'everything is on the table'. Colocation with an adult hospital was an 'important feature', the minister said, as 'the best experts in the world have nailed their colours to the mast on this'. But the Dolphin group could look at other options, even greenfield sites.

'James Reilly is a nostalgic Irish history sort of guy,' according to Tony O'Brien, who was appointed director general designate of the HSE in 2012. 'He still had notions, even then, that this could be a project opening close to the centenary of the state. And he quite liked the notion of building the hospital on the site of the South Dublin Union.'

During the 1916 Rising, a battalion of the Irish Volunteers briefly occupied the South Dublin Union, a former workhouse to the southwest of the city centre, on Easter Monday. It was later renamed St Kevin's and, later again, St James's. A new adult hospital was established there in 1971 and grew around this nucleus in the decades that followed. Now it was a contender for the biggest health project embarked upon by the state that was founded in the aftermath of the Rising.

Reilly rejects any suggestion that the project was being rushed. '2016 was never an issue, not with all the machinations that were happening, and the fact that there was no money, and the Troika in town, and all the other things that had to be done. Remember, there was never a day in the health service when there wasn't some catastrophe or mess.'

~

'Success has many fathers, but failure is an orphan,' John F. Kennedy once said. After the failed planning application, and the political embarrassment it had caused, the Mater's name was toxic in government circles. The often venomous opposition to it in many quarters, the 'northside job' allegation that refused to die and the unresolved planning issues didn't help. The government was determined there would be no repeat of the planning fiasco there.

'There was absolutely no political appetite for the Mater,' according to Tony O'Brien. 'It was always going to be too high. It's an elevated site, too dominant over the city skyline. You couldn't overcome the analysis that An Bord Pleanála put forward, so there was no point.'

'A complete non-runner,' John Martin says of the Mater's effort to win the project a second time. 'It would be full on day one, and it was doubtful that it would get planning permission. An Bord Pleanála's letter for that site was full of red warning signs.'

'We would have to reopen the issue of site selection [if the Mater was picked again], thereby exposing the Government to a raft of medical and constituency lobbying,' Labour leader and tánaiste Eamon Gilmore wrote in his autobiography four years later.

St James's, which had lost out narrowly to the Mater in the previous selection process, was the new favourite, but all the Dublin teaching hospitals were invited to bid.

'It was pretty clear from the day the Mater was rejected that the project was going to be somewhere else,' O'Brien says. 'And given that it had to be colocated with an adult hospital, reasonably proximate to a maternity hospital, all the logic pointed to the St James's site.'

'Frank [Dolphin] had a difficult job, balancing the political pressure with the medical interests,' says Professor Jonathan Hourihane. 'Several of the hospitals who bid had no interest; they just wanted somebody else not to get it. St Vincent's were the only grown-ups who said, "Listen, we're not interested." Everybody else felt they had to play. Some of them were just unrealistic. They brought their whole boards to the meetings, feeling a power play was needed.'

Beaumont Hospital had transplantation and key neurosurgery specialties but, says Martin, 'the problem was that you'd have to knock down the multistorey car park and rebuild it elsewhere'.

The four doctors in the Dolphin group were all professors for whom academic linkages and clinical specialism would have ranked high in importance. 'The merits of the St James's site, especially the academic and specialism integration it offered, were obvious to everyone,' Hourihane says. What people struggled with was: if that was needed as much as was traditionally thought by medical academics? Or would a quick build [beside Connolly Hospital] in Blanchardstown be the better option?

'So it narrowed down to "big, intellectually ambitious in James's and it's a complicated site" – or do you go for a cheaper site in Blanchardstown where there is no academic hinterland but there are green fields?'

While the state's largest hospital was in pole position, there were many other pretenders. Ireland's economy had crashed and many landowners were deeply in debt. The prospect, however dim, of selling a plot to the state offered people a potential way out of their financial problems.

'We got so many offers. I had to turn off my phone,' Dolphin recalls. 'It was 2012, and a lot of people had lost an awful lot of money, had lost their businesses. The country was downsizing. People were driving smaller cars, not spending money.'

People turned up to his office in Waterford unsolicited, trying to promote sites. 'They were hurting, they had land and hoped it would be considered. Others kindly offered sites for free. I didn't entertain them.'

A surprise contender was a site at Belcamp, off the northern end of the M50, where Reilly developed notions of building the children's hospital as part of a wider health and education campus. The minister had recently travelled to China, where he visited a children's hospital and talked to business interests about investing in Irish health education facilities.

'As a group, we were very upset at the outside pressure that was coming on us,' according to John Martin. 'The time pressure was huge, remember. Frank persuaded us to review Belcamp in order to pacify Reilly and provide an objective assessment of the site.'

When its own bid faltered, there was talk of Beaumont proposing a move to the Belcamp campus, which was in the minister's constituency. However, the site was in the flight path of Dublin Airport, effectively killing its prospects. Beaumont later threw its weight behind the bid by Connolly Hospital.

Reilly says he took a 'cursory' look at Belcamp, but it and Blanchardstown would have meant building a new adult hospital alongside a children's one. 'Look at all the trouble we'd had with the children's hospital – when would we ever have got the money to do that?'

The National Asset Management Agency (NAMA) offered 11 possible sites for the hospital. NAMA had plenty of fallow lands on its books, having been set up at the height of the financial crisis in 2009 to deal with the loans given by banks to developers, many of which would never be repaid.

Its lands included the former Irish Glass Bottle site in Ringsend, big enough to house children's, adult and maternity hospitals – if the money were there to build them. There was also a vacant part of Elm Park on Merrion Road near St Vincent's Hospital, several on the North Wall Quay and a land bank adjacent to Tallaght Hospital.

A NAMA site on the South Circular Road had potential, being close to both St James's and the Coombe maternity hospital. And yet not quite in either campus.

Ultimately, the review group chaired by Dolphin received over 40 unsolicited offers, including: lands at Heuston train station; Noel Smyth's holdings at Newlands Cross; a 200-acre site owned by two farmers between Ballymun and Dublin Airport; eight acres on the Navan Road owned by developers Flynn and O'Flaherty; and lands at the Central Mental Hospital in Dundrum, which was due to relocate to north County Dublin. Generous as these offers seemed, those making them were likely to benefit from any decision to build such a huge project on their lands. Arguably, the cheapest option was to simply renovate the existing facility at Crumlin.

'All kinds of crazy proposals were being made and there was loads of gossip around them,' according to Norah Casey. 'By this point in the economic crisis, nobody could sell anything. This wasn't charity. People smelled a public infrastructure project that they could make a profit on.'

James Sheehan, who, as founder of the private Blackrock Clinic, actually had a track record of building and running hospitals, revived a previous offer to design and build the hospital by the M50 motorway for free. He promised to specify all major equipment prior to starting the build, prohibit alterations during it and include a 'no-variation' clause for the price in the construction contract – three issues that would haunt the project later on. 'Why can we not show the Irish nation that it can be done, and give some glimmer of hope to a battered country?' Sheehan asked in an *Irish Times* article in March 2012.

Basing its approach on the findings of the four previous reports, Dolphin's group decided that colocation with an adult hospital was essential. Trilocation with an adult *and* maternity hospital was deemed optimal.

Colocation with a maternity hospital alone was not on the agenda: 'With an initial 56 days to do a report, and a range of complex factors to be considered, you're not going to reinvent McKinsey by looking at things in a different way,' Dolphin reasons.

Accordingly, the group prioritised colocation proposals with Dublin adult teaching hospitals. 'I remember them arriving with jotters, not the iPads favoured by health inspectors,' according to the head of one non-adult teaching hospital, an unsuccessful bidder. 'We could see immediately they had no real interest in us.'

Dolphin says the group did not entertain lobbying by ministers or anyone else, 'because that would create another world'. Once again, it was clear that no site was ideal. Space and access were issues on some sites. Others required major site clearance, or were not in state ownership. And while Connolly Hospital in Blanchardstown was found to offer 'practically limitless scope for further expansion', the adult facility was a secondary hospital and would need substantial investment to bring it up to the breadth and standards of the main Dublin teaching hospitals.

'There is logic to building on a greenfield site. It is clearly easier to do. But this wasn't just about building a hospital; it was building a colocated hospital. Connolly couldn't tick the big boxes. It had plenty of ground but it didn't have the specialties,' says Tony O'Brien.

Building the children's hospital anywhere other than beside a major adult hospital meant that an adult hospital would have to be built there eventually, he says. 'There weren't the resources to do that or the need, so it was never a runner.'

'The four medics involved were absolutely clear that colocation with an adult hospital was the number one criterion,' says Martin. 'From a planning point of view, it came down to either St James's or the Coombe.'

For Reilly, watching from the Department of Health, once Belcamp and Blanchardstown were out of the running, 'that left St James's as the obvious place for the hospital. The Mater had bells and whistles but James's had more specialties, allowing for more kids to be looked after.'

The Mater launched a rearguard action to make up lost ground.

One member of the Dolphin group recalls an 'extraordinary' meeting with Mater executives before they submitted their report, at which the hospital threatened to seek a judicial review: 'We got the sense from the medical politics that there was an awful lot of prestige attached to getting this project.'

What Hourihane calls the 'intellectual' and 'integration' options swung the argument towards St James's. But given the concerns about access to a new hospital, the National Ambulance Service was asked to test journey times. There were negligible time differences in accessing St James's, Connolly and Tallaght from locations across Ireland.

The Dolphin group decided St James's best met the criteria for colocation, because it had the broadest range of specialties and excellent research and education infrastructure.

Still, and ominously, the group noted that the proposed site at St James's was the smallest of the teaching hospitals, 'with some drawbacks in terms of site suitability'. The site offered was 'not without planning risk'.

Dolphin goes to great lengths to emphasise that his group did not pick the site for the hospital, but rather provided the criteria or 'groundwork' on which the minister could base a decision. 'It was not in our mandate to select a site. We were tasked with reviewing the planning issues that led to the Mater's failed application, to consider alternative options and to assess factors like clinical best practice, cost, timelines and risk.'

'Our job was to detail the pros and cons of each location.

The government would decide where the hospital was going,' explains another member of the group. 'The feeling of the group was somewhat split, I would say. If you were a Martian and had just come to Dublin, you'd go for St James's straightaway; it was punching above its weight compared to the other teaching hospitals. But there were people [on the group] who felt the Coombe could have been the right place. Connolly had all the attraction of a greenfield site. As for the Mater, if it didn't work the first time around, it wasn't going to work a second time – that was the general feeling.'

What about the issue of cost, in particular the extra expense of building on a congested site such as St James's, already occupied by various buildings? The group had tried to compare the relative merits of urban versus greenfield locations, and arrived at the conclusion that it would cost about 25 per cent more to build in the city.

'In making the decision to pick St James's, it would have been understood [by government] that this site will be more expensive to build on,' says Dolphin on this point. 'The decision made was to prioritise the clinical synergies [between St James's and a children's hospital].'

At the time, he says, perceptions of the cost involved were 'nowhere near where it ended up'. The focus was on the money spent at the Mater, then estimated at about €40 million, and whether some of this could be recovered. Little attention was paid to the potential for significantly increased costs arising from a cramped location such as St James's.

The group submitted its report to the minister in June 2012, without ranking the various bids. 'It was obvious what our thinking was,' says Martin. 'A careful reading of the site assessments would have made it clear which were in the running and which were not. We were very clear that the decision was one for government, which had to balance such factors as the best medical outcomes, capital cost and planning risk.'

Still a decision was postponed, as Reilly asked two of the group's members, Simon Clear and John Martin, to do a further assessment of the planning issues for each proposal.

Speculation raged as the government appeared to procrastinate. Summer passed without any decision on getting the project back on course following the planning refusal the previous February. According to *Irish Independent* political editor Fionnán Sheahan, the race for the facility was 'neck-and-neck' between St James's and Connolly Hospital, with the Coombe in third place as an 'alternative' and the Mater in fourth.

'It was already clear that it was going to be at St James's,' Tony O'Brien says. The HSE began identifying lands it owned near the hospital in Dublin 8 into which services then on the land intended for the children's hospital could be decanted.

Yet in government, the result was not entirely a foregone conclusion, amid concerns over planning issues at St James's and the extra cost involved in moving to a new site.

One sobering consideration for government was that completion of the project would be delayed by at least two-and-a-half years if the Mater was not chosen, according to the Dolphin group's analysis. The additional cost of moving the hospital to another location was estimated at €120–140 million. This was a sizeable additional cost at a time when building the actual hospital was estimated to cost about €650 million.

Connolly was located in the constituency of ministers Joan Burton and Leo Varadkar, both of whom had lobbied for that site. For it to be brought up to the required standard to host a children's hospital, it would have to be merged with Beaumont. Specialist adult services would have to be transferred to it from the Mater, St James's and other hospitals – a scenario those hospitals were likely to resist.

Civil servants weren't keen. 'This would require the full collaboration of the clinical community and other Dublin adult acute hospitals,' according to a cabinet memo on the issue, obtained under freedom of information legislation. Because beefing up Connolly would require 'very significant additional capital and revenue investment', a decision on siting the new children's hospital there would have to be postponed to allow time for a 'comprehensive business evaluation'.

Tallaght would also require substantial investment if the children's hospital was put there, according to the same memo, and this too would entail pausing the decision. But postponement was the last thing on the government's mind, given how anxious it was to accelerate a landmark project. The hospital had to be finished during its term of office, which was due to run to early 2016 at the latest.

In the final days before a decision was announced, the smart money was on the hospital being sited at the Coombe. With worries persisting about the amount of space available at St James's, this had emerged as a compromise proposal. Government leaders were said to be 'agnostic' as to where on the St James's campus the project was built, so long as it went ahead with as little 'trouble' as possible.

Colocation with a maternity hospital alone had been ruled out, but then the compromise option seemed to gain traction. The Coombe bid, enthusiastically promoted by its master, Professor Chris Fitzpatrick, came near to the ideal of trilocation of the children's hospital with an adult hospital and a maternity hospital, as recommended by the Dolphin review group. At their nearest, St James's and the Coombe are about 600 metres apart.

Twenty acres of vacant land were available beside the Coombe for the hospital. While it wasn't colocation with St James's, services such as human resources, administration and payroll could be shared.

'From a purely planning/building facility point of view, the Coombe site was preferable. It was bigger than St James's,' says John Martin. 'But it didn't offer strict – corridor to corridor – colocation with an adult hospital. Close and all as it was to St James's, this still would have required ambulance transfer. You couldn't wheel a sick mother up Reuben Street and across the Luas line – that just wasn't on.'

Earlier in the bidding process, it had suited St James's to have two irons in the fire. Should the plan to site the children's hospital at the western end of its campus founder due to the space issue, there was always the option of building it down the road at the maternity hospital. But now that Ireland's biggest hospital was favourite to win the project, it was determined to do so on *its* terms.

'The Coombe wasn't the prize possession St James's was looking for in their bid,' Fitzpatrick says. 'We were simply an enabler to help them win the project.'

The amount of land St James's originally offered for the children's hospital was too small, Martin had concluded. But it was encouraged to cede land earmarked for a maternity hospital, thereby reducing the planning risk.

Fitzpatrick says a government aide called a person closely involved in the Coombe bid a few days before the decision was announced to ask if it could be named 'a St James's plan'.

'I agreed to this as the Coombe had offered the plan to St James's at the start of the process,' he says. 'We had no interest in owning the plan or winning the competition. We just wanted to get the hospital built – colocated with an adult hospital and a maternity hospital.'

However, St James's wasn't interested in sharing anything. 'Nobody in St James's was buying the arguments being made by the Coombe about colocation. There were too many issues around the [Coombe] site,' says a source in the adult hospital. 'Up to the weekend before the decision was made, the Coombe felt they had it. But at no point had St James's entertained the Coombe bid.'

'There was nonsense talked, such as getting a monorail to run from the Coombe to the St James's site, so the two hospitals would be connected. But part of the site the hospital proposed using wasn't the Coombe's to offer,' says Jonathan Hourihane, a member of the Dolphin group. 'It was never really a runner.'

Dolphin says the Coombe's bid was attractive and had potential, but there were issues with land ownership and site acquisition costs. Issues that would have taken precious time to resolve.

'We would have had to buy the site, much of it anyway, whereas the HSE actually owned the St James's site,' Tony O'Brien points out.

In October 2012, the planning experts, John Martin and Simon Clear, came down in favour of St James's as the location for the new hospital. Their report was published as an addendum to the Dolphin group report that month.

In November, over 100 days after receiving the Dolphin report, the minister called a press conference. Members of the Dolphin group were told a decision had been made and they should turn up for the photographs. 'We didn't know who had got it until the last moment,' one recalls. 'Then we walked into the Dáil, and we could see pictures on the monitors, so we knew the result.'

I ask Frank Dolphin if he thinks the process of selecting St James's was fair. It was 'the best process for the resources, capability and time we had,' he replies. 'I doubt anyone, anywhere, would come up with a better report. We had no consultancy or research teams supporting our work. We were working through numerous previous reports against the clock. We did our work with the best of intentions and with the best of will, to get the hospital building back on track.'

Criticisms of the St James's site that overlook the importance of the clinical advantages provided by colocation with the adult hospital are 'simplistic,' he says. 'Did we do our work with the best will and intention? Absolutely. Did we come up with the best offering to the government at the time in the circumstances? We did. Am I happy with the treatment of our report in the media and subsequent decision-making? No.

'In 2012 we did not think that it would take to 2017, five years on, before it even started. Our vision of the building was a lot less complex than the one that was built.'

Dolphin says his group interviewed children who were long-term patients in hospital, and asked what was important to them. 'Colocation was important as they got older, views and vistas were not important to them. Good care, breakout areas, space for their parents and space for teenagers to hang out – they were important. I don't think any of us were looking for an iconic building.'

Did he have doubts about the decision to put the hospital in St James's? 'My personal opinion was never asked,' comes Dolphin's terse reply.

At the press conference, Reilly announced St James's as the new location for the children's hospital. 'In these difficult times the new hospital can be a beacon for all of us,' he said, before promising that it would be built by the end of 2017, or certainly by early 2018. This estimate was to prove very optimistic.

St James's, Ireland's largest and fastest-growing hospital, had won the largest health development in the history of the state.

The government told the hospital to allocate additional land on its campus for the children's building so its height didn't exceed seven storeys. By doing so, and allowing for a lower building than had been proposed on the confined Mater site, the risk was reduced of the project being scuppered again at the planning stage.

Reilly declined to say how much the new hospital would cost. But he did acknowledge that St James's cost estimate of €484 million was 'very tight' and said other costs would be involved. This estimate was 'written on the back of a very modest envelope', a source claimed to me at the time. According to the underlying cabinet memo, obtained under freedom of information, the figure 'appears likely to be an underestimation of the final cost in that certain elements of building and commissioning the hospital may have been omitted (for example, in relation to the ambulatory care centre, design team, inflation and lack of risk provision)'.

Cabinet was, effectively, approving St James's as the site for the new hospital despite that hospital seriously underestimating its cost and in the absence of any proper financial examination by the civil service or a cost–benefit analysis. But then the bid by Connolly Hospital was similarly underestimated, the memo notes, not that this counts as justification.

At least the project was up and running again after all the lost time. €360 million was to be provided for the hospital in the capital budget and €200 million was to come from the sale of the National Lottery. But now the economy was recovering fast and construction costs were soaring. An opportunity had been missed to start building while Ireland was in recession, when it could have been done most cheaply. There was also the extra expense involved in moving to a new location. And two-thirds of the money that had been spent on developing the hospital at the Mater would have to be written off.

The term of the development board, which had worked for years to advance the project at the Mater, expired that December, a month after the St James's announcement was made. After five years, members had nothing to show for their efforts.

'The children's hospital should have been the most rewarding thing to do,' Norah Casey says, 'but it turned into the most dispiriting project I have ever been involved with.'

12

'This will never be right'

'The single worst decision undertaken by any government in the history of the state.'

Blackrock Clinic founder Jimmy Sheehan on the decision to locate the national children's hospital at St James's

'This will never be right.'

Retired Crumlin hospital consultant Roisin Healy, veteran opponent of plans to locate the hospital at the Mater and, later, St James's

Thick fog blanketed Ballinamore as Fin Breatnach pulled in to the Leitrim village after a long drive one Saturday morning.

'Be there at 11.30,' his contact had told him, 'and we'll have your money.' It was now the appointed time and there wasn't a soul around in the pub where he was due to meet the fundraising committee. Minutes passed before a shadowy figure materialised on the border village's main street.

'Who told you 11.30, doctor? They'll be along, don't worry. They're all down in the pub,' the man told the visitor from Dublin. 'The other one.'

An hour went by, and then another. Breatnach traipsed in and out to his car nervously. Mobile phones were in their infancy and his, big as a brick, was connected to the battery, with an amplifier in the boot. An oncologist, he was on call that weekend and needed to stay in touch constantly with his hospital in Dublin should an emergency arise with one of his patients.

Around half past one, his contact wandered in along with the rest of the committee. They were still thirsty; the handover of the money would have to wait. It was nearing two o'clock before he was introduced to the group, and asked to say a few words. More speeches followed; may as well sit down again and listen, he thought to himself.

What little light there was in the day was draining away as he finally left. Driving off, Breatnach saw the fog hanging thicker than ever. He got stuck behind a truck carrying a load of offal. The stench was overwhelming; he couldn't overtake for miles.

But it didn't matter; he had the cheque he came so far for, the aggregation of all the sums raised by a small community for sick kids over the past year. His patients, the young children with cancer, could continue to be treated for another while.

'They will live with me for ever,' Breatnach, now a sprightly 78-year-old, says. 'Those memories of fundraising from tiny communities across the country.'

He quickly segues into another yarn. 'There was the time I went down to Enniscorthy to collect a cheque from the women's mini-marathon group who raised funds for us every year. This enormous woman came over to me and said, "Doctor, would you like a dance?"

'And I said, "Of course."

'"Country and Western only," she tells me. So we're in the middle of a conversation and the dance is going full tilt and all of a sudden, I'm lifted in the air. She carries on talking to me, not a bother, and puts me down. Fantastic.'

Breatnach retired early, burned out after 14 years working single-handedly as Ireland's first paediatric oncologist, continuously on-call, in Crumlin hospital. Having set up the Children's Cancer Fund in 1982, he spent many evenings, weekends and holidays fundraising to build a haematology/oncology department, as one didn't exist. It and a bone-marrow transplant unit opened in 1991, entirely paid for by charitable donations.

Fundraising also paid for an upgrade to the radiology department at Crumlin, the country's first CAT scanner for children, surgical lasers and essential staff members for many years. This was the reality of children's medicine in this era; next to no funding was available from government.

'We knew you'd raise the money,' a senior Department of Health official told him much later.

Retirement took the man from the hospital, but not the hospital from the man. For more than a decade, Breatnach has campaigned ceaselessly against the siting of the new children's hospital at St James's. 'Throughout my professional life, my focus has always been on what is best for the children and their families,' he says. 'That focus hasn't changed now that I'm retired.'

Roisin Healy, who worked for many years in the intensive-care departments of Crumlin and Temple Street, has also spent much of her time post-retirement campaigning against the project.

'I can never forget all the nights I spent in Temple Street in particular,' she tells me. 'You look into the eyes of a sick baby, you see the way the baby looks at you and you say, "Kid, my contract is with you. I am going to look after you." That has always been my motivation.'

Since the project was awarded to St James's in 2012, the two doctors have fronted the campaign against that decision through a variety of groups, including the New Children's Hospital Alliance and Connolly for Kids Hospital Campaign. Countless hours of their retirement have been spent lobbying politicians, attending planning hearings, organising demonstrations, speaking to the media and endlessly trying to unpick official arguments. Until recently, Healy continued to archive their petitions, planning objections and critiques of official reports on a dedicated website whose domain name was confusingly similar to that of the development board's.

Theirs has been a David versus Goliath campaign, as their disparate grouping of doctors and parents of sick children faced off against the massed ranks of the political and public service establishment. They often seemed to win the arguments – most of the many people I have talked to for this book think the hospital should be located near the M50 – but were never able to affect the direction of travel of the project.

Their opposition became increasingly quixotic as hundreds of millions of euro were poured into the site at St James's and it became clear that no one in officialdom was for turning. But even today, with the hospital built, the pair still hanker for the project to be relocated to their favoured location beside Connolly Hospital in Blanchardstown and for the Rotunda maternity hospital to be relocated there too.

Breatnach and Healy have no quibble with the principle of consolidating children's tertiary services in one hospital, nor with the idea of colocation. But if children's, adult and maternity hospitals cannot be trilocated – and this ideal looks a very long way off, anywhere in Dublin – they fervently believe the essential colocation that should take place is between a children's hospital and a maternity hospital, rather than a children's hospital and an adult hospital.

Where, they ask, is the evidence showing better outcomes for children from the colocation of adult and children's hospitals? 'This claim is not supported by a single scientific paper,' Breatnach asserts, correctly.

Absence of evidence is not evidence of absence, of course. Juxtaposition may well yield benefits, but the design of studies to test such a complex relationship is a difficult proposition. Logic suggests that children may get access to more specialised services where children's and adult services are near to each other. Colocation may also help with the transition from adolescent to adult services – more than 80 per cent of children treated in children's hospitals have chronic diseases and end up transitioning into adult services.

But to Breatnach's point, there are no research papers showing that sick children do better when their hospital is colocated with an adult hospital. In contrast, there are clear findings that the colocation of children's and maternity services can result in better outcomes, thanks to faster access for newborns to specialised paediatric care and a reduced need for ambulance transport in emergencies. As Breatnach says, 'The critically important colocation is with a maternity hospital, with scores of studies demonstrating improved outcomes as a result.'

Because of the way hospitals are configured in Dublin, newborns requiring emergency treatment must be transported by ambulance from maternity hospitals to children's hospitals. Over many years, this neonatal transport programme has developed in quality and frequency, without a single in-journey fatality occurring. But Breatnach and Healy take no assurance from this, claiming infants can suffer injuries in even the shortest of ambulance journeys.

Now 82, Healy remains steadfast in her opposition. 'My overall feeling is that this will never be right. Forget about everyone going crazy trying to fit everything in. Make a proper plan for children and maternity at Connolly, along with an upgraded adult hospital, and move there in 20 years. Then leave this building for St James's to use.'

Jimmy Sheehan likes lists. The author of pamphlets such as 'Twenty-Four Reasons Why it is not Appropriate to Build the Children's Hospital at St James's' and 'Fifty Things I Would Do if I Were Minister for Health' is also not shy about voicing opinions on the health service.

The soft-spoken Kerryman has been a health entrepreneur for almost 70 years. Trained as an orthopaedic surgeon, and holding a PhD in engineering, he co-founded the Blackrock Clinic in 1986, remortgaging the family home to help pay for the lands on which it was built. Its success spurred him to build the Hermitage Clinic in west Dublin and the Galway Clinic.

A committed Catholic, he runs all his hospitals with a strong religious ethos. His business success made him the public face of private medicine in Ireland for many years and a prominent critic of HSE inefficiencies. In 2005, he offered to rebuild Crumlin hospital on land donated by a developer near the M50 but he says this proposal was never seriously considered.

When St James's was chosen as the location of the new national children's hospital in 2012, Sheehan re-entered the fray. 'I felt it was the wrong site and would be fraught with problems. A huge mistake was being made,' he tells me.

He joined forces with Breatnach, Healy and Jonathan Irwin (who had previously opposed the Mater plan) in the New Children's Hospital Alliance, campaigning for the project to be transferred to a greenfield site in Blanchardstown. The group's brochure is filled with brightly coloured maps and mock-ups of a potential six-storey children's hospital located by a lake across from Connolly Hospital and adjacent to the M50. The cover is emblazoned with a quotation from Pope Francis' *The Joy of the Gospel*: 'Realities are better than ideas.'

Unique among opponents to the St James's project, Sheehan has extensive experience in building hospitals. His clinics were built quickly – the Blackrock Clinic went up in 12 months, the Galway Clinic in 15 – to simple designs. He has seen how much his hospitals have expanded, often very quickly after they were built, how often parking and other requirements were underestimated initially and how quickly expensive equipment and designs can become obsolete.

'You have to design it down to the last plug socket,' he explains.

'There can be no late changes. And you need to commission the hospital while it's being built, not when it's opening.' Commissioning is the testing of a facility's equipment, systems and protocols to ensure they work safely and effectively before patients are admitted.

'To build the new all-Ireland children's hospital on the St James's site would be the single worst decision undertaken by any government in the history of the state,' he told An Bord Pleanála in 2015. 'The care of our children will be compromised for future generations and there will be no turning back or ability to correct this fatal error.'

His warnings fell on deaf ears. 'People pooh-poohed my ideas.' He got no hearing at all. 'We spent a year trying to meet Enda Kenny, but he wouldn't see us. Only the [rural] independents supported us. That's why none of the political parties are up in arms about this; they all backed St James's. I never really understood why.'

Now 86, he wonders if his 'Blackrock image' – his association with private medicine – explains why his warnings were ignored. 'People felt I had a vested interest, when I was offering my services for free.'

Talking to Sheehan, I am struck by how much of the advice he has given over the years ultimately became relevant at the children's hospital, such as the need to sign off plans and to specify equipment before construction begins, for example, or to stick to a simple, modular design. Should we be worried, given that he is now predicting the allegedly €2.24 billion hospital will end up costing €3 billion when legal costs are settled?

Time has caught up on Sheehan, as well as Breatnach and Healy, whose website lies dormant. But in their hearts, they remain sincerely convinced they were right on the children's hospital all along.

Noel Smyth reckons he has spent 'thousands of hours' lobbying to build a new children's hospital, initially in Crumlin, then west Dublin and ultimately on any greenfield site acceptable to the government.

Smyth sought to shift the project away from the city core on numerous occasions, but was unsuccessful each time. At first, his plan was to rebuild Crumlin hospital on a site he controlled near Tallaght. Later, when official policy had switched to a single national children's hospital to be built at the Mater, he canvassed again for a move to Tallaght. And when the project was shifted to St James's, he tried once more to have it moved to the M50.

As one of Ireland's best-known solicitors at the time, with a reputation for dealmaking and an astute eye for public relations, Smyth represented many of the country's leading builders and developers, and later became a property player in his own right. Another devout Catholic, he named his house in south Dublin Lisieux Hall, after the French town where St Thérèse spent most of her life.

His involvement with the children's hospital dates back to the early 2000s. 'I had a friend who was an anaesthetist in Crumlin hospital, who told me what a terrible mess the place was then. So I offered to help.'

Smyth went to see the archbishop of Dublin, Desmond Connell, who expressed a wish to have the hospital rebuilt for the Church. Smyth explained that while a Catholic-owned hospital 'wouldn't work in today's world', a facility run by an independent trust of governors would prevent government from 'interfering'.

He sat down with officials from Micheál Martin's Department of Health but got a frosty reception for his idea of a privately funded, non-profit hospital. Smyth's view was that since Crumlin was not publicly owned, the state should have to pay 'reasonable value' for the services provided by its replacement.

'It was an interesting meeting. The concept I was explaining to them was beyond what they thought possible. In particular, the idea of an independent hospital was anathema to them. They were keen for the rebuilding of Crumlin to go ahead but I wasn't interested in building a hospital for the state. That didn't go down well.'

Smyth concluded that the civil servants could be convinced but it would take time. Deciding he needed a site of his own to show people, he purchased the 32-acre plot off the Naas Road he had been offering for the project and set up a trust to own it. Building a children's hospital there would cost €150 million less than at the Mater, he claimed.

His consortium developed a proposal for a children's hospital with almost 600 beds. He also suggested building a maternity hospital on the same site with 400 beds. The European Investment Bank was willing to loan his charity €600 million, he said, pending a full appraisal. The plan was for the children's hospital to charge the HSE for the services provided on a fee per item basis.

Over time, he proposed building further 'profit centres' on the campus, such as a 24-hour laboratory and a college for wealthy students from China and the Middle East. 'This would allow the campus to become self-sufficient for funding,' he says now. 'The department suggested a public-private partnership but I said that wasn't going to happen. My ideas fell on deaf ears.'

When the McKinsey report in 2006 proposed a single national children's hospital, colocated with an adult hospital, Smyth bid for the project on the basis that Tallaght Hospital was a mile away from his lands. Again, he was unsuccessful.

Smyth continued to canvass ministers even after the Mater was selected. In 2007, he offered to build the hospital at cost price at the Mater or any other location preferred by government.

He appeared finally to be making progress in 2010 when Philip Lynch, the chairman of the National Paediatric Hospital Development Board, met him and walked the lands at Tallaght. By now, Smyth estimated the cost of his new hospital at €300 million and promised it could be ready within 30 months of planning permission being granted.

Lynch had begun to have doubts about the Mater site and was actively investigating Smyth's project but he was sacked by minister for health Mary Harney in October 2010 for deviating from the Mater plan.

By the time the Mater site was refused planning permission in 2012, the Tallaght lands were in NAMA because of the economic crash. The government, if it were minded, would have to pay for their use. Smyth says he continued to make numerous offers to build the project 'anywhere' in the years that followed.

'It's a pity it has ended up the way it has,' he says. 'What I tried was done out of the best of intentions. It didn't work – *c'est la vie*.'

The plan to locate the national children's hospital at the Mater, and later at St James's, has had many media critics, but none so forthright and dogged as Pat Kenny.

The issue is personal for the veteran broadcaster, whose daughter was successfully treated for childhood cancer over 20 years ago. 'I know what it's like to look after a child who is neutropenic and at risk of infection, and has to be brought to hospital by car rather than taking public transport,' he says. 'So I could see how much epic nonsense was being talked about in relation to the hospital.'

Kenny says he understands the 'desperation' that led the parents of sick children to support the bids of the Mater and then St James's in the belief that this was the fastest way to get the much-needed hospital. In the end, though, as he points out, 'it didn't get built quickly'.

Traffic concerns loom large in his assessment of the various hospital sites. When his mother was in St James's for rehab after a fall, Kenny found himself visiting her on a motorbike to beat the 'appalling' tailbacks into the hospital car parks.

His first interaction with the children's hospital story dates back over two decades, long before the Mater was chosen as the location. A landowner in west Dublin who was offering his property to host the hospital suggested that Kenny have a closer look from the air.

'The land was beside a park and he wanted to build the hospital in a quarry there. This fellow had a chopper so he flew me and the cameraman over the site. While there was lots of fresh air, I remember, it didn't jump out and recommend itself to me as the best place for a hospital.'

The landowner then offered to fly Kenny over other potential sites, but a trip over the Mater wasn't possible due to the proximity of Mountjoy Prison.

Kenny says the selection of the Mater for the children's hospital was 'bizarre' in planning terms: 'What was proposed was a carbuncle on top of the existing hospital. The location might have been a runner but not with that design. It was nonsense and it smacked of political chicanery. I think UCD, too, saw it as their chance to get a toe in the door, to match Trinity's links with St James's.'

After the Mater was rejected on planning grounds, St James's was selected. Kenny says Leo Varadkar promised him on air that a planning application for a maternity hospital on the site would be lodged at the same time as the application for a children's hospital. That didn't happen.

'Trilocation of an adult, children's and maternity hospital – that was the vision. But that's gone out the window at St James's – there isn't room for a maternity hospital there now. Then you had the sewer that had to be moved at enormous cost, and the epic traffic in Dublin 8. It was illogical.'

On his radio shows, Kenny consistently championed Connolly as the best location for the hospital, much to the annoyance of those planning the new building at St James's.

'Blanchardstown [Connolly] is doable, there's plenty of room,' he says. 'The adult hospital needed upgrading, true, but just think what we could have done with all the money spent at St James's.' Though he does add: 'This was before the M50 became the car park it is now.'

Even now, he wishes the political establishment would admit 'we made a bit of a bags of it' and do things differently. Like Breatnach and Healy, he suggests giving the new building to St James's for its use and getting 'someone like Jimmy Sheehan' to build a new children's hospital in Blanchardstown.

13

High Stakes and Lowballs

'When we saw the site, we thought – in a way – what's the fuss about?'

Children's hospital architect Benedict Zucchi, making light of the challenges of building on the St James's site, September 2014

'There is no perfect or ideal site as such, each will have their own strengths and weaknesses.'

Planning inspector Tom Rabbette, in his report on the planning application to build the children's hospital at St James's, April 2016

In November 2012, the month the decision was made to build the new children's hospital at St James's, I visited Temple Street for *The Irish Times*.

Dublin's oldest surviving children's hospital was marking its 140th anniversary. 'It looks every minute of it,' I wrote.

> A maze of narrow corridors and dark and dingy stairs, it looks like a cross from the worlds of Charles Dickens and *Alice in Wonderland*. Staff and parents alike daily toil up steps, past the 'mind your head' signs and the cracked windows, and through a rabbit-warren of passages and rooms.

The lift doesn't reach the top floors so children have to be carried up to the Top Flat ward for sick babies. Any youngster unable to climb the steep stairs likewise has to be carried up to the school and the playroom.

Top Flat has just one adjacent toilet for 14 beds and no work area for staff. Patient notes are written up on a small ledge. Every available area of floor and wall space is used to store or hang equipment and parents staying with their children have to make do with armchairs or thin mattresses placed on the floor.

This is the reality of children's medicine in Ireland today; a similar story could be told at Our Lady's Hospital in Crumlin or Tallaght children's hospital.

The replacement of Temple Street and the other dilapidated children's hospitals was inching forward again. However, the backdrop to this plan was very different from the days of planning for the Mater site, with the *vroom* of the Celtic Tiger supplanted by the misery of economic collapse. More than ever, the new children's hospital stood out as a beacon of hope. Here was a project for the nation to rally for, while all around it chaos reigned. The political pressure to get it back on track after the Mater planning debacle was enormous. Visible signs of progress were needed after all the years of delay.

This rush by ministers to get started would have fateful consequences, though these weren't obvious at the time. And the hurry was probably wasted, given that the new government's term was due to end in early 2016. The dream of successive governments

– to open the flagship project in time for the centenary of the 1916 Rising – had already been long extinguished.

Meanwhile, James Reilly was proving a loose cannon politically. Barely a year after entering office in 2011, his name appeared in a debt defaulters' list over a business deal involving a nursing home. While he survived a motion of no-confidence over health cuts in September 2012, his Labour junior minister, Róisín Shortall, resigned that month in a dispute over primary-care centres. Nicknamed 'Calamity James' by the media, he had the misfortune to get stuck in a lift while on official business and, on another occasion, to fall over in a playground.

To minimise any unwanted surprises, Taoiseach Enda Kenny and Tánaiste Eamon Gilmore had both involved themselves personally in the decision-making process for the children's hospital, before it came to cabinet. 'They didn't have a vested interest, but they wanted what was best for children and the country,' Joan Burton, who succeeded Gilmore as tánaiste, tells me. 'Ultimately, doctors enormously influenced where the hospital was located, and most of them wanted it in the city centre or the southside.'

For once, given the past history of the project, it stood to St James's advantage that it was in a constituency with no government minister. This time around, there could be no accusations of pork-barrel politics.

The move to a new location meant that most money spent on the children's hospital at the Mater – then estimated at €33 million – and a previous €16 million spent planning the transfer of Temple Street to the Mater, was dead money. Scores of architects, engineers, lawyers and other professionals earned handsomely for designs that, for one reason or another, went nowhere. And this waste loomed large in public debate at a time when the government was under pressure to watch costs.

St James's was still viewed as risky in planning terms. Access was better than at the Mater, but not by much. The lands on which the new hospital would be built were occupied by a chapel and other buildings. These would have to be demolished and existing services decanted elsewhere. All of this would take time and money.

Looking back on coverage at this time, it is surprising how little of it concerned the cost of the project. The change of location had done nothing to diminish opposition, with 'Anywhere but the Mater' quickly morphing into 'Anywhere but St James's'. Those in favour of building the hospital on a greenfield site tended to highlight the benefits of fresh air for children and easier car access for their parents, rather than lower cost. But now that St James's had been selected as the location, the state was going to have to devote serious resources to the project. And yet no one seemed to know for sure how much it would cost.

Had St James's lowballed the cost of building the hospital? 'It does seem so,' says Leo Varadkar. 'But nobody in the early days questioned that it might cost €500 million, because that seemed like a lot of money.' He laughs: 'It doesn't seem so much now.'

Lowballing can happen in the planning of infrastructure, he says. 'Often the government prepares a national development plan or multi-annual capital plan. There's a financial envelope into which ministers try to fit as many projects as possible. That incentivises departments and agencies to lowball their estimates so that they are more likely to get into the plan. But the projects cost what they cost, and the plan gets updated every two or three years anyway.'

'We paid no attention to the cost estimates that the hospitals put in,' says John Martin, a member of the Dolphin review group. 'But we did a lot of work on the difference in cost between greenfield and brownfield [previously used] sites. Brownfield [as at St James's] could cost up to 25 per cent more than a greenfield site. So the government would have been very aware from day one that if they were going for St James's versus Connolly, there was a significant trade-off in cost.'

Should the Dolphin group have interrogated the St James's estimate more?

'No,' Martin replies.

Because people were going to lowball anyway?

'Yes. Every site was different, so we didn't pay any attention to the costs different hospitals put in.'

'No great account would be taken of an individual hospital's estimation of the cost,' then HSE director general Tony O'Brien says, though he acknowledges 'there probably wasn't sufficient time given to fully considering' this issue. 'There was a strong desire to make progress quickly and not allow the political process to burn more time. I understand that. They wanted the project to be live at the time of the centenary [of the state]. That was an emotional outlook.'

Notwithstanding their name, the parents in the New Crumlin Hospital Group rowed in behind the new location, but medical staff at Our Lady's were less supportive. Forty of its consultants called for the hospital to be sited at the Coombe, physically attached to the adult hospital by a corridor. A campaigning group led by consultants from Crumlin, the New Children's Hospital Alliance, said it would not support any proposal that did not involve colocation with a maternity hospital. Every year, the group pointed out, up to 500 seriously ill children required ambulance transfer to ICU units in children's hospitals. This would continue to be the case until colocation with a maternity hospital was achieved.

The Alliance, when it rowed in behind Connolly Hospital's bid, claimed that children could be scared if they had to attend a hospital in Dublin's inner city. 'The kind of environment around city-centre locations can be frightening for children. You have to provide safety and security for them,' according to Dr Trevor Duffy, clinical director of Connolly Hospital. Building the hospital in Blanchardstown would save €130 million, compared to the next cheapest bid, he predicted.

Meanwhile, as I wrote at the time, children continued to be treated in rundown hospitals across the city. Given the ongoing delay in building the new children's hospital, tough decisions were required about renovating existing facilities for the shorter term.

The development board set up to build a new children's hospital was over six years in existence, and not a brick had been laid. Now government had formally approved the project at its new location, but even then, work was slow to get underway.

Over a year earlier, in June 2011, Labour minister for public expenditure Brendan Howlin and Fine Gael minister for environment Phil Hogan had announced upgrades to their local hospitals in Wexford and Kilkenny respectively, before the HSE board even knew about them. 'The people of Wexford want, demand, and are going to get the highest standards of healthcare,' Howlin had said, when revealing that his hometown hospital was getting a new emergency department. Neither project was a priority in the HSE capital plan, and the money spent on them was originally earmarked for the children's hospital. Was it any surprise that progress at St James's was so halting?

Still, Enda Kenny, approaching the end of a lengthy political career, was keen for the project to advance. The story of the children's hospital was to be converted from a political negative into a positive.

Reilly left vacant the 12 seats on the hospital's development board when the members' terms ended in December 2012 and suggested it might be abolished. In February 2013, he appointed six of his officials to manage the project on a temporary basis while he rethought its governance. By May, the schedule for building the hospital had slipped back a year. Costs were said to be €650 million, of which €150 million was to come from still unspecified philanthropic sources.

That month, the minister made a technical announcement that was to have profound consequences: the National Paediatric Hospital Development Board (NPHDB) was to be restructured to make its sole focus the design and construction of the building. This 'build board' would 'oversee very tightly the actual building and project management' of the hospital, the minister promised.

In place of the doctors and health officials on the previous board, Reilly intended to fill this version with experts in building and construction.

The newly reconstituted board would 'ensure that we end up with the best hospital, in the quickest fashion', the minister explained. It would also ensure that 'all due precautions are taken in negotiating with those in a position to influence the eventual outcome'.

Reilly said he wanted no repeat of the problems encountered in the past when different hospitals were brought together 'and took a long time to bed down'.

Construction industry veteran Tom Costello was appointed chairman of the new board in August 2013, working part-time for up to two days a week. From Mayo, Costello had been managing director of John Sisk builders for 13 years, but left in 2012 in the aftermath of the economic crash. In a lengthy career, he had worked on some of Ireland's biggest building projects – the Aviva Stadium, Croke Park, the Dundrum Town Centre and the Mater Hospital. He promised a 'robust cost control' approach that would help bring in the project on budget.

The new board, heavily weighted towards engineering and architectural experience, included solicitor Tim Bouchier-Hayes, who led the construction department of McCann FitzGerald for 15 years. Planner John Martin, who had served on the Dolphin review group, and architect-planner Karl Kent were appointed to ensure that the planning application for St James's did not fall foul of An Bord Pleanála in the same way the application for the Mater had.

'It was very thinly resourced in the early days,' Martin says.

'There were no planners or architects employed by the board, so it depended entirely on us and the effort we were prepared to put in. Karl and I were both retired. I put in three to four days a week on the project, up to the time planning permission was given.'

A separate body, the Children's Hospital Group (later Children's Health Ireland/CHI) was to be established to merge the three existing children's hospitals over time. Dr Jim Browne, an engineer and president of NUI Galway, was appointed as its chairman. The appointees to this new group included representatives of the three existing children's hospitals, several doctors from outside the Republic and figures from business and law. Pointedly, no doctors from the children's hospitals were invited to join.

CHI was, effectively, the client of the development board. In time, it was planned, it would become the operator of the hospital, with responsibility for integrating the existing facilities and their staff. The NPHDB – the development board – was responsible for building the children's hospital and its satellite centres.

Reilly says he was determined the 'mayhem' that accompanied previous hospital mergers in Dublin, which he remembered from his time as a GP, would not reoccur. 'It was important that the hospital board [CHI] focused on bringing together all the professionals and on controlling demands, while the 'build board' got on with building a highly technical, huge hospital.'

The government's chief procurement officer was on the 'build board' while HSE Estates were represented on the hospital board, he points out.

In the most general sense, CHI was about people and processes and the development board was about the physical elements.

CHI was independent from the HSE, yet it was funded by the Department of Health through the HSE.

It sounded good, and no one doubted that reforms were needed, particularly greater expertise in construction. But an additional layer of oversight was being created. From this point on, it was unclear who was ultimately responsible for the project. 'The pantomime horse was in two parts now,' says a source familiar with the process. 'One end wanted to build the best possible hospital but had no direct responsibility for costs. The other was supposedly in charge of costs but had no influence over the build. It was a recipe for disaster.'

Eilish Hardiman, who had been chief executive of the development board until she left to become chief executive of Tallaght Hospital in 2011, returned in September 2013 as chief executive of CHI. While this brought much-needed continuity to the project, Hardiman was no longer directly involved in the hospital's constuction.

The project received a boost when Crumlin hospital gave its 'categorical' support for locating the hospital at the western end of St James's – this despite many of its doctors favouring other options. The times were finally changing; a Catholic children's hospital in Dublin was aligning itself with St James's and its academic partner, the once exclusively Protestant Trinity College Dublin.

Reilly obtained cabinet approval for two urgent-care centres, in Tallaght and Blanchardstown, to deal with the less serious cases that might otherwise overburden the new hospital. 'It was important to get both centres to open before the children's hospital so that parents would be in the habit of going there,' says John Martin. 'There was no way the big hospital at St James's could have handled all the demand in the Dublin area.'

Leading architectural firms from Ireland and overseas bid to design this prestige project but there was further delay in their consideration. A board spokesman said this was because of the need for 'very rigorous financial evaluation' of the bids. 'It is essential to get the detail right now at project planning stage,' he added, 'so as to minimise problems later in the project when it is on-site [subject to planning permission].'

The more closely the site was examined, the more problems emerged. A large sewer serving the southwest of Dublin ran directly under the site and would have to be rerouted, allegedly at a cost of €18 million. Not to mention the church and graveyard mapped on the site, and the need to move numerous existing services at St James's offsite.

Other challenges loomed. Builders were lodging 'unsustainable low-cost bids' to win contracts, and then trying to recoup the money through 'active claims management' during construction, a report presented to the board in February 2014 warned. 'This has led to little or no collaboration, poor value [and] dispute resolution and a lack of cost certainty,' according to the report on procurement strategy.

With so much time lost up to this point, the board was under pressure to work as fast as possible. Procuring the project in the normal manner would mean that construction could not start until the full design of the building was complete – and this could take years given how complex it was.

What if there was a better way to procure construction of the hospital? What if this was broken into two stages? In the first, work could begin on-site while the final design brief was being finalised, thereby saving time. The report estimated that the project could be delivered a year or two earlier through this process.

But it warned that this approach was 'more aggressive and would place added pressure on the design team'. While the cost of the project – known as the guaranteed maximum price – could be agreed with the contractor, it would be 'poor quality'.

At least the general requirements for floor space, operating theatres and rooms had been worked out previously for the hospital planned for the Mater site. 'It was now a question of transferring that information to a very differently shaped building,' John Martin says.

In July 2014, I was the first journalist to visit the St James's site, which I walked with John Pollock, the boots-on-the-ground project director for the development board. 'The new national children's hospital could break the Government if it fails,' I wrote.

> Poppies, buddleia, acres of car-parking and a few clapped-out hospital buildings – there's little to indicate that this land at the back of St James's Hospital may soon become the biggest building site in the State.

We're standing on the roof of the old Hospital 7 in St James's – the patients have been moved elsewhere – and I'm trying to imagine the creation of a high-rise, world-class hospital for the sick children of Ireland arising from this jumble.

John Pollock, project director for the team building the national paediatric hospital, has his own vision of how this project will evolve and he's convinced we're in the right place. 'This is a cracking site in the middle of the city. In agricultural terms, it's a small farm, a quarter mile from one end to the other.'

Years after a new national children's hospital was first mooted, this is as far as the project has got. There's a boring machine taking soil samples and a few billboards promising to 'work together for our children's future'. Sick children and their parents shouldn't hold their breaths. Real progress has to await the granting of planning permission – if it is granted – over a year hence.

The design team will be confirmed shortly, but Pollock's team has done the preparatory work. They've surveyed the site, the traffic situation, even the bat population (there is none). The buildings on site are being emptied and a 'multifaith centre' is being built to replace a soon-to-be-demolished nineteenth-century chapel.

After many false starts, most notably the failed planning application for the Mater site, the hospital is now on track in the right location, Pollock maintains. 'This site is large. That's the lesson we learned from the Mater; it didn't fail because of traffic or medical issues, [but] because of over-densification.'

Because this site is twice as large, Pollock believes a seven- to eight-storey building will accommodate the new hospital, compared to the sixteen-storey behemoth planned at the Mater. That should pass muster with the planners, he says. Unlike the Mater, the current project has the full cost of €650 million committed by the government.

Pollock spent thirty years in civil engineering and when the downturn hit, he shifted his work to the Middle East, building medical facilities in Saudi Arabia. That experience is now being brought to bear on the government's flagship project; if it doesn't work out, and planning permission is refused at the end of next year, it could end up scuppering the government itself. That's not a scenario Pollock envisages happening, as he responds to the arguments that have been thrown up in opposition to this site.

The Drimnagh sewer, which runs under the land, will be left in place and built around, he says, though the design team will make the final decision.

'It's two pipes. To listen to Jonathan [Irwin, chief executive of Jack and Jill charity, a firm opponent of the site], it's like moving the port tunnel.'

A more substantial concern is traffic. There are already almost 1,500 parking spaces in St James's, most of them for staff, and another 1,000 spaces for patients of the children's hospital are envisaged. Yet access is tight and the approach roads frequently clogged.

Pollock blames morning and evening traffic jams around the existing hospital on the large numbers of staff commuting to and from work. 'The business of the HSE and of hospitals is healthcare, not car parks. I'm not saying it's the easiest site to get to, but it's not about a building, it's about children's lives and clinical outcomes. The idea we would protect so much valuable land just for staff parking doesn't make sense,' he says.

There will be adequate parking for patients, so that sick children can make it to the hospital unimpeded. Pollock makes the point that, currently, 'people are not dying on the roads' because they can't get to the adult hospital.

The other main criticism of St James's is the absence of a maternity hospital on the campus, though the Coombe is down the road. Pollock says the vast majority of patient movements from maternity hospitals to children's hospitals are pre-planned, rather than emergency situations.

St James's is home to thirteen medical specialities, against one in the Mater and two in Beaumont, he points out, so children will benefit from the proximity of high-class care in areas such as plastic surgery, burns and cardio-thoracic medicine.

Another acre or so, currently a car park, is being ringfenced for a maternity hospital, though it is likely to be years before this project gets off the ground.

The aim is to complete building the children's hospital 'by the end of 2018'.

That month, July 2014, saw a government reshuffle. Reilly, fresh from a humiliating U-turn on medical-card cuts, was demoted to the Department of Children.

Today, he says he is happy to defend his actions on the hospital project. 'The decisions we took were based on sound international advice and my own gut realisation that a) we were looking at building a children's hospital, and there was no question of adding on anything for the foreseeable future and b) that kids and their families come first.

'I cannot explain the astonishing increase in money since but I suspect there have been changes to the original design. That always escalates costs.'

The hospital was one of '30 to 40 things going on at the time' in his department. 'There was an [overall] picture. Did I go through every single detail of every single room? Am I qualified to decide whether something was right or not? That's why you have architects, medical specialists and so on.'

Rising star Leo Varadkar was installed as minister for health in July 2014. With budget cuts imminent, the abolition of the HSE on the cards and its headquarters at Hawkins House 'falling down', the children's hospital project wasn't one of the new minister's most urgent priorities, according to a senior official at the time.

From his time training as a junior doctor in Crumlin, before the project was to be located at St James's, Varadkar knew the medics campaigning to move the project to Connolly Hospital. Personally, he favoured a greenfield site in west Dublin, and if that was in his constituency, all the better.

But he says he gave the campaigners a 'wide berth'. The decision had been made and he felt opponents such as Jonathan Irwin were excessively negative towards government. 'I'm sure had it been on a greenfield site, it [the cost] would also have overrun, but probably not as much, nor for as long.'

One of the new minister's first actions was to request the files for the children's hospital and to speak to Frank Dolphin. It was, he realised, too late to reverse out of building at St James's. As he wrote in his autobiography *Speaking My Mind*, published in 2025: 'The decisions had been made by government, and returning to site selection and design would have set us back years on an important infrastructural project that was already well behind schedule. I pressed on.'

Any doubts were superseded by a desire to get on with a project that had been delayed so much, and to create a 'statement piece' at St James's, according to the department official. 'We'd had the IMF [International Monetary Fund] and the Troika – very little bread and no roses, and penury the order of the day. So the feeling was "let's go the extra mile" with this hospital. Let's give the country something people can be proud of, something that will last the test of time.'

The contract to design the children's hospital was awarded to O'Connell Mahon Architects (who had designed the earlier, aborted project at the Mater) and international partner BDP (Building Design Partnership) in Manchester. Leading engineering consultancies Arup and O'Connor Sutton Cronin and quantity surveying firm Bruce Shaw (renamed Linesight in 2016) joined BDP on the design team.

British architect Benedict Zucchi of BDP was appointed to lead it. The company had a strong record in designing children's hospitals, including Alder Hey in Liverpool, known as 'the children's hospital in the park'. Then under construction, Alder Hey was, ironically, on a greenfield site. It would be completed for a fraction of the cost of its Irish counterpart.

All hospital projects are inherently complex – in fact, they are the most complex projects architects have to design, Zucchi told journalists at an event in September 2014. 'When we saw the site, we thought – in a way – what's the fuss about? We've worked on projects that were more challenging in terms of sites. Hospital projects in Britain; the new children's hospital in Brighton, for example, which is on a much tighter site. We're used to working through complex projects and dealing with those kinds of issues.'

Funding seemed assured; the government was now providing €450 million in capital funding and another €200 million was to come from the €405 million sale of the licence to operate the National Lottery. Varadkar promised that a maternity hospital would be built beside the planned children's hospital 'within the next decade'. He even suggested outline planning permission would be sought for the maternity hospital at the same time as the children's hospital, but this idea was quickly abandoned as impractical. 'I was told, and accepted, that if they had to do that as well, it would slow down the children's hospital,' he says.

'Whether I was right to accept that advice or not, I don't know, but I did. In retrospect, I am sure now that we should have gone for trilocation from day zero and if I knew then what I know now, I would have insisted on it when I became minister for health,' he says.

Yet the size of the project was starting to cause problems across the cash-strapped health sector. Varadkar said the government had enough money to build the facility but not to equip it. He complained there was 'no provision' for IT for the hospital unless his capital budget was increased. At St James's, the adult hospital was forced to defer a planned expansion of cancer facilities because its campus could not cope with two major construction projects occurring at the same time.

John Martin, the retired planner and member of the development board, chaired a planning subcommittee set up to steer the project safely through An Bord Pleanála. He focused on the building's height and traffic, two of the issues on which the Mater planning application had foundered. The height issue was tackled by doubling the site area. 'And we tried to be as respectful as we could to local residents. The hospital didn't come out right to the road; it had these little fingers. We were very careful about overlooking,' Martin explains.

Traffic was a huge challenge, he says. 'Coming in the main gate of St James's then, you'd be in a queue of cars right up to the parking areas. We had to convince An Bord Pleanála and Dublin City Council that we could make the entire campus – the adult and children's hospitals, and a future maternity hospital – work for traffic.'

Winning over the planners meant promoting public transport and reducing the share of people arriving by car. It helped that

St James's had the best public transport links of any Dublin hospital, with a Luas line running alongside the hospital. But with thousands of staff expected to work in the hospital, just 325 parking spaces were being provided for them, along with 675 for visitors and patients. The latter figure was a multiple of the admittedly insufficient 230 spaces then available in Crumlin, Temple Street and Tallaght combined. Unsurprisingly, though, the proposed provision wasn't large enough to silence arguments over parking, which would continue for years.

Road access was tight, so another recurring concern was ambulance access to the children's hospital. But then ambulances already served the adult hospital at St James's, for the most part without problems. 'The National Ambulance Service told us that when they get to a patient, the first thing they do is stabilise the person,' Martin says. 'If they have done that successfully, the transport element becomes less critical.'

The design for the new hospital was unveiled in April 2015. The proposed building was oval-shaped on its most prominent upper floors and featured a children's 'therapeutic garden' on the roof and an inner courtyard. At its highest point, it rose to seven storeys – less than half the height of the building proposed for the Mater site that had been rejected by An Bord Pleanála.

The hospital was designed to be child-friendly. The design team said they aimed to give the hospital a 'memorable quality that captures the imagination of children and gives it a unique sense of place'. The building would incorporate a simplified orientation with different areas clearly distinguishable from one another, 'ensuring that the space is less daunting and more in keeping with the scale of things familiar to children, like houses and trees'.

There were 380 single inpatient rooms, with 42 beds in a critical-care unit and 18 in a neonatal critical-care unit. In addition, 93 day beds were being provided, more than twice what McKinsey had recommended. The hospital was now scheduled to open in 2020 – a slippage of two years in two and a half years.

Varadkar described the design as 'breathtaking' and said he was confident it would get planning permission. But a predecessor as minister for health had also been confident when the Mater planning application had been prepared years earlier.

The design, with its internal 'floating garden' and barrel-vaulted roof of profiled zinc, did indeed seem better integrated with its surrounding, admittedly cramped, environment than at the Mater. The 1,000 parking spaces were out of view in a double-basement car park. There was also a helipad for emergencies, on the roof of a four-storey building facing the adjoining Luas line.

Architect Benedict Zucchi identified the main challenges as 'scale, complexity and speed'. The bottom three floors of the building would be built from grey granite 'in the civic tradition of Dublin', he told the *Architects' Journal*, while the top three floors, built above the roof garden, would be covered with metallic panels. The oval shape of the building was designed to respond to the design of formal gardens elsewhere in the city.

Zucchi said it had been refreshing to work on the procurement process, with the contractor responsible for building the designs set to be appointed separately. 'There has been a real focus on the quality of the project and we are going to see the project through to the end, working with the contractor.'

Four years after the first oral hearing into the project at the Mater, a fresh oral hearing into the children's hospital project at St James's got underway at An Bord Pleanála in November 2015. The location was different, but many of the same issues – and faces – reappeared.

The new application was mindful of the planning mistakes made at the Mater. This time, the design was more compact, the site available was bigger and the consensus in the medical community behind the project was stronger – though after all the delays, this support often took the form of a 'just get on with it' sentiment.

With every passing year, the need for a new hospital had grown more urgent, as facilities in the existing children's hospitals had become more dilapidated and waiting lists had lengthened. The new hospital offered slightly more inpatient and day beds (473, compared to 432 then in the three Dublin children's hospitals), more operating theatres (18 against 12), and more MRI machines (seven against two-and-a-half). By providing more specialised care to a higher standard, it offered the hope of better health outcomes for children.

All manner of concerns were ventilated at the ten-day oral hearing, from vermin to the local swift population, but the central issues were access and traffic. Heavier search-and-rescue helicopters operated by the Irish Coastguard would not be able to use the helipad because it was on a rooftop, the hearing heard, though light Air Corps helicopters were projected to use it up to 200 times a year. There were claims that the area where the entrance to the hospital would be was prone to flooding.

Despite universal agreement on the need for a new hospital, St James's was being opposed for many of the same reasons put forward against the Mater. The arguments around access, traffic and parking were rooted in a view that the development should be designed around the needs of car drivers over other users. In this view, St James's was just as damned as the Mater for being an inner-city location with limited space and traffic-congestion issues.

Once again, the 'Dublin versus the rest' urban–rural arguments played out, as opponents pleaded for the project to be relocated to the M50, said to be more easily reachable by car from all parts of the country (though poorly served by public transport).

Capacity issues also emerged. The hospital would not be able to meet the demand for emergency treatment without many children being encouraged to seek treatment elsewhere. Up to half of all children requiring urgent care would be treated in the two satellite centres in Tallaght and Blanchardstown, the hearing was told.

The plan was for children with fever, rash, vomiting and diarrhoea, or sprains and fractures, to attend an urgent-care unit. These centres would have observation beds but no inpatient beds. Children requiring emergency care involving life- or limb-saving treatment – for example, meningitis, pneumonia, multiple fractures or a collapsed lung – would be treated 24/7 in the new hospital.

Hundreds of very sick newborns would still need to be transported by ambulance every year from a maternity hospital to the children's hospital until a maternity unit was built at St James's. While this wasn't ideal, doctors pointed out that no child had died while being moved during the 14 years the neonatal transport programme had been in existence.

By the end of the ten-day hearing, the smart money was on the development getting the green light from planners. However, in February 2016, An Board Pleanála delayed a decision on the planning application for another three months, pleading the complexity of the issues before it – though the fact that a general election had been called might also have been a factor.

Even at this late stage, opponents rallied, commissioning an opinion poll showing that 73 per cent of people wanted the hospital built somewhere else. Meanwhile, the government had by now spent the €200 million windfall from the sale of the National Lottery supposedly earmarked for the project, so a funding shortfall remained.

By March 2016, as the state marked the one-hundredth anniversary of the 1916 Rising, the application remained on the drawing board. 'Once again the project threatens to become a symbol of how Ireland struggles to implement big projects and wastes millions of euro instead of inciting pride over our ability to deliver what the health service needs, when it needs it,' I wrote in *The Irish Times* that month.

By now, the realisation was dawning that a golden opportunity had been missed. 'The time for building the hospital was during the economic doldrums when costs were lowest and the employment it could have provided would have been gold dust,' I pointed out. Costs were projected to rise an extra €60 million on top of the initial €650 million estimate, but I felt that was 'probably only the start of it' based on previous experience with public projects. Construction inflation – set to become a familiar theme in the years to come – was already running at 7.5 per cent, more than twice the rate that applied when previous cost projections were made.

Though all reporting from this period quotes an estimated cost of €650 million, the development board had prepared a preliminary budget of €800 million in early 2014. Something that did not emerge until 2017.

In late April 2016, with the election safely out of the way, An Bord Pleanála gave its decision. Planning permission was granted, subject to 17 conditions, none of them overly stringent.

'There is no other public healthcare site in the State as well served by public transport as St James's,' planning inspector Tom Rabbette commented in his 293-page report. Local road traffic would be affected, he said, but mitigation measures should keep this to 'acceptable' levels.

'There is no perfect or ideal site as such, each will have their own strengths and weaknesses,' Rabbette noted, echoing the words of so many previous reports on the project.

He described the hospital as a long-awaited and much-needed piece of national strategic development that had the potential to adversely impact its environment. However, the proposal kept these adverse impacts broadly 'within acceptable levels'.

The board's decision was welcomed by parents who had long campaigned for the new hospital. 'You can see the zombie parents walking the corridors at night time,' said Louis Roden, the father of two children with cystic fibrosis. 'This will do away with all of that. There will be a bed for the parents in the room with the child.' Families do not just attend children's hospitals, he pointed out, they often live in them.

In retrospect, this was the high-water mark of the project. A site for the hospital had been found and planning permission obtained. All the children's hospitals were finally on board and a good-looking, inspiring design had been finalised. Issues around cost were mere rumblings at this stage.

Varadkar described the decision as 'fantastic news' and made his most extravagant promise yet. Funding for the hospital was in place and 'short of an asteroid hitting the planet', it would be built by 2020.

14

The Most Expensive Children's Hospital in the World?

'Oh God, not BAM.'

Leo Varadkar's reaction on hearing that the Dutch-owned contractor had been awarded the contract to build the children's hospital

'Are we now looking at a project that will cost over €2 billion, which would make it the most expensive hospital in the world?'

An unnamed Department of Public Expenditure official, in a memo to a colleague in the Department of Health

After multiple reports and broken promises, and tens of millions of euro squandered on the failed planning application at the Mater, the way was finally cleared for the project to go ahead.

Well, almost. The development board was 'absolutely terrified' of the threat of a judicial review challenging An Bord Pleanála's decision, according to John Martin. 'It was an enormously complex planning application – a large hospital, two urgent-care centres, the Ronald McDonald accommodation block for parents [funded by McDonald's fast-food chain], a research and innovation centre. If it went to the courts by way of judicial review, we were bunched.'

Martin had spotted a prominent serial litigant on planning issues 'floating around' the oral hearing. There were fears that opponents would play the environmental card to stall the development. Lawyers were briefed to ensure any potential loopholes in EU directives were closed. A court challenge was considered likely.

Yet it never materialised. No legal proceedings were lodged within the requisite eight-week period after the planning permission had been granted. 'We all heaved an enormous sigh,' Martin says.

The task of advancing the project fell to a new government and a new minister for health. Fine Gael lost 26 seats in the February 2016 election and Taoiseach Enda Kenny needed the support of independents to form a minority administration three months later.

Varadkar, perceived by Kenny as an impatient pretender, was demoted to the Department of Social Protection. He seemed unperturbed to be leaving health and the challenges of the children's hospital after just two years.

Twenty-nine-year-old Simon Harris was the surprise choice as his successor. 'The new man's lack of a track record in the area left many scratching their heads over what his appointment might mean for the health sector,' I wrote at the time.

Meanwhile, An Bord Pleanála's unanimous decision to grant planning permission didn't still opponents for long. The Connolly for Kids group again called on the government to change the location, and collected 60,000 signatures in support of its campaign to move the hospital to the M50.

However, Jonathan Irwin, one of the most trenchant critics of the St James's site, while expressing disappointment at the decision, said it had to be accepted: 'We've made our point. We've done our best. We lost. And now we've got to move on.'

In October 2016, at the Oireachtas health committee, Connolly for Kids representative Valerin O'Shea claimed that Harris would be responsible for the deaths of 'many' children unless the hospital was moved to Blanchardstown.

'If a colocated maternity hospital is not built, then it is inevitable that babies will continue to die each year during the planned 100-year lifespan of the children's hospital,' Dr Fin Breatnach had warned in a press statement issued in advance of the committee meeting.

Such dire warnings cut no ice with government and were probably counter-productive. Even those ministers who were sympathetic to the notion of switching sites felt the project was too far advanced to change now. Harris accused campaigners against St James's of using 'offensive' language.

Harris tells me he bought into an existing line on the hospital from officials and leading doctors. 'When I became minister, the site had been picked and the design and planning permission were done but the debate on the location was still going on. So the immediate political decision was: "Are we proceeding?"'

He agrees that construction on a greenfield site would have been more straightforward. 'But the officials and the paediatricians persuaded, convinced, reassured me that all this debate was done with. It was just a case of getting on with the project.'

Though a start to building was some way off, the project was beginning to take practical shape. 'We're at the stage where detailed decisions on the new hospital are being made, such as where to place the plugs in the 6,000 rooms in the new building,' Eilish Hardiman said.

And yet the problems started immediately. Site clearance was delayed. Promised legislation to merge the three existing children's hospitals into a single legal entity failed to materialise. Plans to give the hospital a name dragged on, with 25 options under consideration.

The development board put on roadshows in the Irish embassy in London and other overseas venues, trying to drum up interest in the construction sector to tender for the project. There were doubts whether any Irish firm was big enough to build the hospital on its own, and to handle the complexity of both the site and the building. Officials hoped for joint-ventures between big international contractors and Irish partners bidding for the project.

Under the tender rules, 75 per cent of marks were awarded for price and 25 per cent for quality. But the successful bid on price received 100 per cent of the marks available, while quality was marked on a pro-rata basis. This meant bidders had to aim low. As Martin explains, 'If you won on price, you weren't going to be overtaken.'

One criterion that wasn't taken into account, but would be raised as an issue later, was a contractor's previous record for claims and disputes. The children's hospital, as a public project, was subject to strict state and EU procurement rules. The kinds of side deals that private developers were free to cut with their contractors were not an option here.

Five bidders expressed interest in the tender to build the hospital along with the two smaller satellite centres in Tallaght and Blanchardstown. Four of them progressed to a final shortlist.

The best-known was John Sisk, a leading Irish construction firm founded in 1859. In the nineteenth century, Sisk built churches, banks, hotels and housing across Ireland; in the twentieth, its major projects included Liberty Hall, the Ballymun flats, the Central Bank, Croke Park and Lansdowne Road, as well as shopping centres in Tallaght, Blanchardstown and Dundrum. The company was part of the fabric of Irish life, though it had suffered in the economic crash, when one-third of its workforce was cut.

Over the previous decade or so, Sisk's primacy in the market had come under threat from an upstart rival. BAM Ireland was the Irish subsidiary of Royal BAM, a leading global construction and civil-engineering company headquartered in the Netherlands (BAM stands for Bataafsche Aanneming Maatschappij – Batavian Construction Company). With roots in a Dutch–Irish joint-venture created to build a bridge in Wexford in the 1950s, the company had become one of the country's largest civil-engineering and public-works contractors, building roads, schools, hospital infrastructure and commercial premises across the country. The company was originally a civil-engineering specialist but after Corkman Theo Cullinane took over as chief executive in 2009, the construction side of its business grew considerably, as did its reputation for aggressively chasing new business by bidding low for contracts. The company had won the contract to carry out the enabling works at St James's in June 2016, so there was no surprise that it made the shortlist for building the actual hospital.

The other two bidders shortlisted by the development board were joint-ventures between Irish family firms and big building companies headquartered in Spain: Dragados and Collen Construction; and FCC Construcción and Walls Construction.

The tender for construction of the basement, foundations and main building of the hospital closed in October 2016. It took until the following February for a winner to be announced.

The four bidders submitted multiple boxes of technical information, but each of their money offers was contained in a slim, sealed packet. Once all were submitted, the boxes were opened in the presence of board members, and the sealed packets retrieved.

The packets were opened in the presence of development board members, one of whom recalls the occasion as 'very tense'. BAM Ireland had submitted the lowest bid. Under the rules of the tender process, which prioritised price, the company couldn't lose. It was designated the preferred bidder.

In Ireland, BAM had built the pipeline tunnel for Shell's Corrib gas project in County Mayo and City Gate Park in Mahon, Cork, the largest commercial development built during the recession. It had completed major developments for Google, Intel and Microsoft. But it hadn't built a hospital in Ireland before, or taken on a project of this size and complexity. And while it had a parent company to lean on, there was no joint-venture partner in its bid.

The firm had a reputation for tendering low bids for contracts and then being hard-nosed when negotiating cost changes later on. 'BAM had form,' says Leo Varadkar. 'I remember on hearing they had got the contract having one of those heart-sinking moments – thinking, *Oh God, not BAM*.'

Relations between the company and government had taken a knock a few years earlier when it began legal action after losing out on a contract to build a college campus at Grangegorman. BAM argued that a rival company's successful bid should be invalidated because it was submitted 90 minutes after the deadline, but the High Court rejected its challenge in 2016. Varadkar describes the resulting delay to that project as 'pretty annoying'.

Also, in 2014, the company had been awarded the initial tender to build an events centre in Cork. Taoiseach Enda Kenny turned up two years later for a turning-the-sod photo op during the general-election campaign. However, procurement issues led to delays. Twelve years on, the project is still stalled, amid spiralling estimates of the state contribution and the overall cost.

Despite these flashpoints, the company continued to win state contracts for motorways, courthouses, schools and health centres, and these were successfully completed.

While outsiders perceive a commercially aggressive company, BAM's self-image is that of a price-conscious disrupter in a hitherto cosy construction sector dominated by traditional Irish firms. As the only large construction company in Ireland with a multinational parent, it is in a position to bid competitively for big projects using resources from its headquarters in the Netherlands. Its rapid rise has undoubtedly ruffled a few feathers, while forcing rivals to revise their construction bids downwards. At least some of the complaints made about 'the Dutch company' verge on xenophobia, staffers have complained to me.

For St James's, BAM's offer came in well under the next lowest bid. But its figure was above internal cost estimates, which rather undermines subsequent accusations of lowballing. 'The big shock to us was that BAM were themselves higher than our quantity surveyors had estimated, by over €60 million,' says John Martin. 'That should have been a big warning sign to the board that our cost estimates were skewed.'

The quality of BAM's bid was as high as and even better than the others, according to one board insider. He says the gap with the internal estimate 'raised some concerns but was tiny with hindsight'.

To counteract the rise in costs, the development board had introduced a €70 million value engineering target; in other words, it undertook to save this amount by cutting costs, for example by switching to cheaper materials or removing elements of the design. This gave the impression that the project was staying within its capital budget, when all the indications from the tender process was that it would cost more.

The tender bids were higher than the development board's €575 million estimate of the cost of construction of the hospital building by a range of €61 million to €239 million. BAM's bid of €636 million came in €131 million lower than the next highest bid, from John Sisk. The two other bids, from Dragados/Collen Construction and FCC Construcción/Walls Construction, came in even higher. With hindsight, the wide spread of the bids should also have set alarm bells ringing.

BAM had tendered on its own for the project rather than partnering in a joint-venture after obtaining special permission from its Dutch parent board to exceed the normal threshold applying to such arrangements. And it did so on the basis of an indicated project cost that would quickly be exceeded.

The marriage of development board and contractor had been uneasy from the start. In the first phase of digging the foundations, the development board had hired a firm to count the number of workers on the site. 'That shows you the level of antagonism there was, even in those early days,' Martin says.

It didn't take long for rumours to circulate about rising budgets. Independent TD Mattie McGrath, a staunch opponent of siting the hospital at St James's, claimed the anticipated costs were 'like a runaway train'.

He wasn't wrong. In February 2017, I reported that the overall cost of building the hospital and two satellite centres was now estimated at close to €1 billion.

This was over €300 million higher than the €650 million price tag attached to the project at the time planning permission was sought in 2015 – an increase of almost 50 per cent in two years. And the new agreed figure didn't include the cost of IT systems or equipment, I reported, which were each expected to cost €100 million.

Rising costs in the construction sector, driven by an improving financial outlook, were blamed for most of the projected cost increase. As the economy continued its recovery, building inflation rose from 3 per cent when the project was mooted at St James's, to almost 9 per cent when the building contract was awarded.

The development board's plan to economise came to nothing as inflation surged. 'The approach adopted by the board was value engineering, but it didn't work,' according to Martin. Substituting 'cheaper' solutions, materials and specifications did not save any money, because their prices had risen since the contract with the original, fixed-price items was written.

The outcome of the tender placed the government in a quandary, given the competing demands for spending in health and continuing opposition to the project. 'Building the hospital, and moving the Central Mental Hospital to north Dublin, will consume most of the HSE's capital budget over the coming years, unless additional funds are made available,' I wrote in *The Irish Times*. HSE director general Tony O'Brien, keen to replace clapped-out ambulances and ageing nursing homes, said the service could not afford to build the hospital unless capital funding for the health service was increased.

Against these concerns, there was the tantalising prospect of building Ireland's first super-hospital by 2021. And who wanted the embarrassing legacy of so much wasted investment if the project were to be stopped now?

Varadkar, now minister for social protection but conscious of his legacy in health, pleaded for a longer term view: 'Look at Terminal Two [at Dublin Airport]. It cost a fortune ... but it has worked out really well and will pay for itself over time. The children's hospital is a project that you have to take a one-hundred-year look at.'

But concerns about the potential cost of the new hospital only grew. 'The proposed €1 billion National Children's Hospital in

Dublin will be the most expensive children's hospital to be built anywhere in the world,' I predicted in an article in February 2017, basing my estimate on international data.

The facility was on course to be the second most expensive hospital ever built, I wrote. Only the futuristic Royal Adelaide Hospital in Australia cost more to build, a ranking by architectural data company Emporis appeared to show.

The recently built Alder Hey children's hospital in Liverpool, which had been designed by the same architects planning St James's but was smaller with 270 beds, cost just €330 million, I pointed out. In Finland, the budget for the Nova children's hospital, about the same size as the Irish project, was €500 million – and this included IT and equipment. Something was seriously wrong at St James's.

Around this time, I paid another visit to the site. Outside of a quarry, I had never seen such a huge hole in the ground. From its rim, I could see the machines that were used to create the hole moving around the bottom; from this distance, they looked as small as children's toys. The sides of the hole were lined with curved white curtains of concrete, which dazzled whenever the sun shone. Most bizarre of all was the sight of a small row of local cottages, gingerly perched above this monster civil-engineering creation. I was no expert, but I could see that this wasn't straightforward work.

The contract drawn up between BAM and the development board allowed for below-ground works to begin immediately.

But government approval would be needed before phase 2 – construction of the hospital building – could begin.

This was an unusual kind of contract for a public project, conceived for a specific purpose – to get a large project built faster. Ever since the Mater fiasco, the development board had been under tremendous pressure to make up for the delays that had occurred. But progressing the hospital in the traditional manner meant nothing could happen until a completed design was ready. And this was likely to be a lengthy process, due to the size and complexity of the project.

'We spent a year working out the best procurement approach with the Department of Public Expenditure,' a source tells me. 'The country was just out of recession; the construction industry was destroyed. We figured there was no chance we'd get people to bid to design and build the hospital [because of the front-loaded cost for the contractor].'

In an attempt to make immediate headway, a derogation from the traditional method of procurement was approved. The contract would be split into two stages, or phases.

The first phase was itself composed of two elements. The first covered a full design of the basement works of the project, and the second, a *preliminary* design of the works above ground – the actual building. An overall *indicative* contract sum could be finalised at this point.

In the second phase, a *detailed* design of the hospital building was to be completed, while the first-phase works were under construction. A full bill of quantities priced at preliminary rates during this stage was supposed to produce a detailed estimate of the cost, referred to as the guaranteed maximum price (GMP).

The practice of splitting contracts into two phases had grown in popularity during the Celtic Tiger era, when the economy was stretched to its limits and haste was the order of the day. 'We would design the basement of a building and then do the next bits along the way to save time. It made sense in that environment,' one architect says of this period.

The idea of the two-stage or two-phase contract appears to have originated in a sub-committee of the development board, found favour with the Department of Public Expenditure and the Department of Health and was eventually agreed by all those involved. It wasn't for the want of internal discussion that the proposal was born.

'It was looked at by the contracts committee and the advice received, external to the Department of Health, was that this was the best way to proceed,' says Simon Harris, minister for health at the time. 'It needed to be constructed like that to get the interest of the person who was going to build the second part. It was clear to the officials who briefed me that there was going to be a limited number of people who could build the hospital. And an even smaller number who would be interested in building it.'

So one aim was to lure potential contractors into bidding for the project. Another was to allow work to start early while the detail of later phases was being finalised and agreed. The GMP was supposed to deliver certainty over price. Officials vaunted the new approach for facilitating a quick start, but in time it was to come back to haunt them.

'At this stage, we were in a fantastic place,' a source says. 'The design was well developed, despite what people say. We felt it was 90 per cent accurate, though in hindsight it was closer to 75–80 per cent.'

'We were under the cosh to get things moving, but to do a full design for this enormously complex hospital plus the two care centres was going to be a complex process,' says John Martin, who stayed on the development board for a time after planning permission was obtained.

'They [a procurement subcommittee] recommended it would make a lot of sense to go for a two-stage process. Construction firms were told they could bid for phase A – the underground stuff [basement works] – based on bills of quantities and the plans our design team had prepared. While they were doing that, more detailed plans could be worked up for the actual building. That would save time, it was explained. The contractor could get ahead and start with the underground parts, and we could refine the design for the super-structure.'

Around this time, the talk in construction was of new approaches to procurement based on cooperation. 'You'd tell the builder that if they could get savings, they'd get a percentage of the sum. The extras were divvied out,' says one architect.

The development board wanted such a collaborative approach for phase B in place for the children's hospital, and got approval to deviate from the standard public-works contract from the government's construction contracts committee. 'It seemed to make sense in terms of saving time, possibly going down the collaborative route, and it had approval from a government body,'

John Martin explains. 'From a layman's point of view, the approach seemed to make common sense. We hoped the two design teams would work together and there would be cost savings.'

Construction could start two years earlier than if a traditional procurement strategy had been used, the board estimated. Buying materials this much earlier should allow for them to be bought more cheaply.

'This change was critical to what happened later,' HSE boss Tony O'Brien argues. 'It satisfied the objective of getting the project moving. There was a big focus, for example, on getting the site shuttered with pictures of a future hospital and the name of the contractor and all of that. This was not unrelated to Enda Kenny stepping down [which happened in June 2017] and a desire to get some evidence of this project, given there was a general election in the offing [this didn't take place until 2020]. You had a lot of desire to achieve cosmetic things that would work politically, but which may, with the benefit of hindsight, have complicated the project.'

O'Brien, who was director general of the HSE from 2013 to 2018, says he has 'a lot of respect' for the officials building the hospital. 'But they were taking instructions from the political system as to what they were to build. That system was supported by a department that had no expertise within it. It was not a balanced governance process. They went off and did what they were told to do.'

What happened with the contract was 'no different to your average kitchen extension' where things go wrong, he says; just on a different scale. 'Normally you start with a fairly good design.

You procure a design team [an architect, structural engineer, and so forth], they design the thing, and then you procure a builder to build it. Your design team is heavily involved in the management of the contractor. There'll still be some changes as you go along but you know exactly what you're trying to build before you procure your contract.

'Here, the procurement went a different route, in that they procured on a non fully designed building. They procured on a concept. The building was not yet [fully] designed when they brought the contractor on board, in this case BAM.

'The problem with that is you don't have a fixed reference point to go back to. There always has to be an allowance for changes of some sort but if you're pricing a job that isn't fully specced, you don't have a fixed reference point against which to have the arguments later on.'

And while deals and trade-offs between the contractor and those paying the bills are a normal feature of private-sector builds, in the more rules-bound public sector, this arrangement was to contribute to lengthy stand-offs between the development board and BAM.

Rural independent TDs opposed to the location of the hospital tabled a Dáil motion aimed at forcing the government to conduct a cost–benefit analysis of the already over-budget project. While this was defeated, the project remained mired in bad press.

'Arguments for putting the hospital on the M50 popped up at every forum,' O'Brien recalls. 'Every place I ended up in, answering questions about anything at all, there was always a question about moving the hospital.

'I took a firm line at this point, saying that, once the government had made the decision, we needed to get on and build the thing. The project had been on the books for so long, while people continued arguing about where it should be. I knew the condition of Crumlin and Temple Street, so this wasn't something that could be let go on and on.

'I also made the point that there is no perfect site for the hospital. Let's not let perfection be the enemy of the good.' He adds: 'That's a whole different story to what has happened since in terms of the project management and all that.'

Publicly, Fine Gael TDs accused opponents who raised cost issues of 'scaremongering'. Inside government, however, and at the highest levels of the public service, concerns were rising.

The Department of Public Expenditure demanded to know more about governance arrangements and the future running costs of the hospital. It wanted assurances about the roles and responsibilities of the Department of Health, the HSE, the hospital development board and the Children's Hospital Group.

'Are we now looking at a project that will cost over €2 billion, which would make it the most expensive hospital in the world?' one of its officials asked in an internal memo of the Department of Health.

There was also the challenge of finding the shortfall in funding for the project, after the estimated cost had increased. Would the health service stump up the extra money or would the burden be shared among government departments?

Already, about €60 million had been spent at St James's as the site was cleared, on top of the millions wasted on previous iterations of the project at the Mater. It was generally accepted that this money would be lost if the project was halted.

Varadkar says the government did look at other options by awarding contracts to 'the most economically advantageous offer' – theoretically, a higher bidder – rather than simply on price. But what if the decision were challenged in the courts? And, if a challenge were successful, would retendering be needed?

The attorney general was asked to see if a bidder could be allocated negative points in tender competition where problems had arisen in previous contracts. The proposal never progressed. 'What came back was that in order to impose a negative mark against a contractor, there would have to be actual findings against them, not just someone's opinion,' Varadkar says.

In late April 2017, the Department of Public Expenditure felt it had received assurances from the Department of Health that 'sufficiently robust' governance arrangements were now in place.

Simon Harris, in his formal approvals authorising the development board to engage BAM, warned that additional costs were to be avoided or addressed through reducing the scope of the project. He told journalists that he expected the hospital would be delivered on budget and on time. It was not fair to say the cost of the hospital had 'spiralled', he argued, because extra facilities were now being provided in addition to the basic hospital construction.

In anticipation of disputes over cost, mediation and conciliation mechanisms were put in place for the project. The development board engaged an 'employer's representative' (a member of the design team) to administer day-to-day relations with the contractor on its behalf. Where disagreements persisted, they could be appealed to a standing conciliation mechanism presided over by an arbitrator. If this failed to resolve issues, the courts beckoned. Works would continue while this machinery was sorting out issues.

That month, ministers made the decision to go ahead with building the hospital, based on a 'definitive business case' pricing the cost at €983 million. This was an umbrella sum comprising €571 million for construction and equipping and €412 million for other project work, such as decanting services, training facilities, VAT, IT, integrating the existing three hospitals and provision for risk.

All previous figures relating to the cost of the building were mere estimates; this global sum was supposed to deliver certainty. From now on, there was no turning back.

15

A Relationship Made in Hell

'It is unbelievable that in the space of two years the projected cost of delivering the national children's hospital has more than doubled from €650 million in 2016 to a projected €1.4 billion now.'

Labour health spokesman Alan Kelly, December 2018

'We always expected that the price would rise as a result of construction inflation but the latest increase is way beyond what we had ever anticipated.'

Leo Varadkar, December 2018

The design of children's hospitals around the world has changed hugely in the twenty-first century, and no one knows this better than US architect Bill Mead.

Mead reckons he has designed at least ten children's hospitals across North America over the course of a long career, starting in the mid-1990s. He is now in active retirement in Massachusetts – 'I could say I was busy but does pickleball count?' he quips when apologising for being hard to reach. I have got in contact with him in order to learn something about modern trends in the design of children's hospitals internationally.

Almost all the hospitals Mead has designed were colocated with an adult hospital, he tells me. The prioritisation of children's needs and a recognition that they benefit from a healing environment are the key factors driving reforms in the way hospitals are built and services provided for them, he says.

'In the original model, you went to the door of the hospital with your children and handed them over the threshold. Staff said, "We'll call you when they're better." Now, families move in with the child if possible until they get better.

'Today, it's recognised that children need a special place of their own, an entire environment suited to their needs. Accommodate their families in the healing process and they get better faster.'

Working alongside doctors and families on a new children's hospital in Rhode Island in the 1990s, Mead learned that things needed to be done differently. 'The doctor can't just stand in the middle of a big room and be able to see all the patients anymore. Sorry, that might be good for the doctor but it's not so good for the kids.

'We used an arrangement of small-scale "neighbourhoods" of beds, more adapted to children and their size, so they weren't overwhelmed or overstressed. Everything about the experience of visiting the hospital, starting with the drive into the car park, was adapted to make people more relaxed and less nervous, so they would heal faster. It caught on and now we're doing it for adult patients.'

The resulting hospital costs slightly more, he says. 'The units are smaller, families need to be accommodated too, and more money is spent on interior design – sculpture, patterns on the floor, that kind of thing. The infrastructure is basically the same but it's a more playful environment.

'The hardest thing was battling with the doctors for control of the patients. You'd have an intensive-care doctor opposed to single rooms, saying, "I can't take care of my patients this way; I need to be able to stand in the middle of the room." So you had to have someone, a high-level administrator say, who could push back and say, "That may be good for you, but it's not going to be good for the patients."'

Single-bed rooms require higher staffing levels, but Mead says there are 'lots of studies' showing that patients get better faster with this arrangement, thereby saving money. And while children are sociable beings, and interaction between them is to be encouraged, single-bed rooms 'work better' overall.

As between building in the city or on the periphery, he says greenfield sites are clearly easier and less expensive. 'It's much more complicated building on an existing campus, but you also have to look where the demand is. And getting to those campuses mightn't be easy for staff as well as patients.'

As for whether a children's hospital should be built up or out – vertically or horizontally – Mead believes it depends on the site. Most US children's hospitals are located in dense urban environments with little space, he says, because 'that's where the patients are'.

'Distances are shorter when you stack it vertically, but that's probably more expensive unless you include real-estate costs. Here in the US, we've looked at moving all these hospitals out of the city to a greenfield site but the cost is such a joke that no one does it.

'The challenge is when you start conceptualising the project you have no idea what the challenges will be. You can't anticipate it all, and if you did, the contingencies would be so high that nobody would ever start the project. You start hopeful you won't run into so much and inevitably you run into just as much.'

Meanwhile, the demands for space keep changing, as does the technology available. 'It's impossible to keep up with the technology when it takes so long to do these things. The budget and the schedule have to be free-flowing, dynamic things, worked on by fresh teams of architects and builders in the same room, figuring out the problems.

'Healthcare is so complicated. You need really smart people designing and building, who are willing to work together and then hurdle all the challenges that come up in every single project. I don't know how we did any of it.'

It is clear to me from talking to Mead that the national children's hospital, as it has been designed, is ticking some important boxes – colocation with an adult hospital, child-centred design and services, for example. The hospital isn't unusual in being built in a cramped downtown site but – and this is a big but – the successful realisation of such a project is dependent on intelligent and open-minded collaboration between architects and builders working together.

After all the delays, the August 2017 signing of contracts to start building at St James's was a time to celebrate the new vision being created for children's health. As long as Grafton Street and as big as the Dundrum Town Centre, the hospital promised single en-suite rooms for every patient, with glorious views of the Dublin mountains. There would be ample sleeping accommodation for parents and acres of rooftop gardens in a sheltered, child-friendly design. The vision for the hospital embraced the latest in technology; the project team planned 'automated delivery systems' to deliver children their food, hospital-wide wifi and the first fully truly digital public hospital in the state, using electronic health records, patients apps, automated logistics and integrated building systems.

The plans for the new building reflected the principles followed by Mead and others in designing modern children's hospitals across the world. Chief architect Benedict Zucchi talked of a 'choreography of public spaces and the progression from the front door to the threshold of individual clinical areas to break up the perceived scale and make the hospitals feel as "open" and free of conventional corridors as possible'.

This, he said, would be achieved by 'maximising the relationship between inside and outside' to take full advantage of daylight, views and access to gardens. 'These might seem obvious architectural strategies, but in the past they tended to be given a low priority. A "therapeutically designed environment" has proven benefits for patient wellbeing and recovery times.'

Most rooms would have garden views, Zucchi pointed out. 'Proximity to the outside, in contrast to the traditional deep-plan approach of the older generation of hospitals, also underpins the drive for improved sustainability, with increased potential for natural ventilation, particularly in wards.'

Many doctors I have spoken to proclaim the therapeutic benefits of fresh air, ample play space and engaging views in helping sick children to heal.

Others believe these claims are overstated. 'This idea that all Irish medical healthcare for children has to be done in beautiful places,' says paediatrician Jonathan Hourihane. '"Give them an iPad and a slide!" Children only need that when they're well. Children who are sick just need carers and their parents.'

Hourihane points out that when children with long-term illnesses – the patients mostly likely to spend extended periods in treatment – were surveyed for the hospital, 'they said they didn't care about trees and views. They just wanted their mother or father and their doctor'.

The grander vision that imputes therapeutic value to good architecture won out in the design of the hospital, where it was married to the political desire to create a legacy building. 'We created a vision for the hospital that cost money,' says one of those centrally involved at this stage. 'Architecturally, it was best in class – stone-clad, sustainable, with daylight available everywhere and outdoor terraces. This is a huge civic building, so the atrium needs to be a grand space. Yes, we could have done it cheaper, but we're a wealthy country.'

With construction of the building due to start, new problems arose. Local residents took a High Court case claiming their homes had been damaged by ground works on the site, leading to cracks and 'movement'. The case was to continue for four years, on and off. Proceedings were withdrawn, then re-entered before going to mediation. In 2021, a confidential settlement was reached.

Next up was a row over fire safety standards. In June 2017, a high-rise fire broke out in Grenfell Tower in London, killing 72 people and prompting a review of fire regulations in high buildings internationally. Dublin City Council demanded that sprinklers be installed throughout the children's hospital building, not just in the upper floors, basement and canteens. The development board appealed this condition, arguing that its existing design exceeded current fire standards.

In October, An Bord Pleanála found against the development board. The sprinkler system had to be redesigned to cover the entire hospital, adding €16 million to the cost of the project. The total cost overrun had reached €60 million, and the estimated final cost was now €710 million.

That month it was announced that the facility would be named Phoenix Children's Hospital Ireland. The name 'aptly represented the level of renewal and regeneration under way in paediatric healthcare in Ireland today', or so Children's Health Ireland announced on completion of its 'comprehensive naming process'. The new name was 'a symbol of hope and optimism and positively represents our vision for the future'.

CHI claimed the new name was chosen by staff after nine months of consultation, but doctors at the existing children's hospitals were immediately critical. Phoenix, given the suggestion of rising from the ashes, was an ill-conceived name for a hospital dealing with children with very serious conditions, one pointed out. After all, it wasn't that long since Crumlin hospital had been convulsed by a scandal over the retention of children's organs, which were later incinerated. The proposed new name might serve as a constant reminder to families of their loss, another doctor said.

A more pressing problem soon arose. Phoenix Children's Hospital, a well-known paediatric centre in the US, expressed concern about the 'unavoidable likelihood of confusion' between the two hospitals. Very quickly, it threatened legal action. CHI's proposal, which cost €40,000, was dropped.

What's in a name? The failed attempt to find one for the children's hospital was only a minor sidebar in this story, but the manner in which it was handled hardly inspired confidence in the wider project and the way money was being spent.

The project did secure a European Investment Bank loan of €490 million, the biggest single investment the bank had made in Ireland. A community-benefit programme was set up to ensure that local people in Dublin 8 got employment on Ireland's biggest building site, and there was talk of the hospital driving urban regeneration in an area that badly needed it.

In June 2018, barely a year after construction of the hospital had begun, John Pollock travelled across Dublin city centre for a regular meeting of the Children's Hospital Project and Programme (CHP&P) board in Hawkins House, the Department of Health's headquarters.

This group, chaired by the department's secretary-general and including the director general of the HSE, had been set up by government a year earlier to provide high-level oversight of the project. Its brief was to ensure that the hospital was delivered against agreed parameters for timeline, scope and funding. Members were also supposed to sort out any bottlenecks and ensure the seamless integration of the three existing children's hospitals – while getting on with their presumably busy jobs running the rest of the health service.

The development board was now reporting to the CHP&P board on a quarterly basis and to a lower-level body known as the steering group each month. This latter body had already discussed concerns over rising costs but this was the first time Pollock was bringing bad news directly to the top of the public service.

The hospital was facing 'cost challenges and pressures', Pollock told senior officials, due to construction inflation, 'gaps' in the design and delays, minutes of the meeting record. There was also 'seeming resistance' on the part of contractors to engage in securing greater value – a reference to the development board's failed attempt to make savings on the project, for example by using cheaper materials.

At previous meetings in the spring, Pollock had mentioned that pricing agreements with contractors were 'unsatisfactory' and that 'pricing discrepancies' between quantity surveyors and contractors were being referred to an independent adjudicator. It was clear that something was amiss.

The contractors were also feeling the strain. BAM's Dutch parent board expressed concern about the scale of the project as it was now emerging, and the challenges of finding qualified workers to build it. In a memo to the employer's representative on the project, Royal BAM warned that full employment in Ireland and the development of other large projects at the time might place 'impossible strains' on the resources needed to complete the project.

At this point, the detailed design of the hospital building was still underway. From this was supposed to come the detailed cost estimate or guaranteed maximum price. But internal and external circumstances were changing and, with them, BAM's assessment of what it was due.

By August, the construction budget was running €191 million over what had been agreed a year earlier. As well as the sprinklers and the failure to make promised savings, there were changes to specifications – doors, lights, partitions – and an increase in the quantities of materials needed.

This was only the start of the bad news. This figure did not include VAT, pay increases and 'hyperinflation' as defined in the contract. BAM needed longer to complete the work and it had submitted an additional €200 million in cost claims. These it attributed to inflation, the need to pass on national wage rises and mark-ups for mechanical and electrical specialists.

'As a board, we were shellshocked when the claims started coming in,' says John Martin. 'We couldn't believe the price escalation.'

The board was trapped. The contract was designed so that if a guaranteed maximum price wasn't agreed, it could part company with BAM. The contractor could leave with what it had earned and the board could retender.

But, Martin says, this was a 'non-starter from the beginning. I don't know how anyone put any trust in that. It would have been extraordinarily difficult to get another builder to take over the project.'

In October, the project steering group discussed options for reducing the funding deficit, including scaling back the design or reallocating money from other health developments.

This revealed another major flaw in the contract. There was

no point in replacing expensive design items because the lower rates in the contract applied only to items originally tendered for in 2016. Swapping out glass balustrades, say, with cheaper perforated metal alternatives, would cost as much, if not more, at current prices, the officials discovered. Planned savings could not be achieved.

That autumn, concerns about cost creep began to spread more widely. For months, I had been hearing the rumours but my enquiries were stonewalled. No firm information was yet available, I was repeatedly told.

Details finally emerged as the issue wended its way towards cabinet and the first leaks occurred. The estimated final cost of the hospital was now €1.4 billion, Martin Wall and Pat Leahy reported for *The Irish Times* in December 2018. In just six weeks, the officially cited cost had grown by €400 million. And the bill was continuing to increase as more design changes were made.

The necessity for design change was built into the process because of the two-stage contract. 'The hospital couldn't have been fully designed at the time of tenders. That process was formulated to allow for refinement,' says John Martin, who left the board in May 2019. 'Given the gap between the business case and the cheapest tender, we knew that costs would go up.'

Yet, while increases were anticipated, the rise from €980 million to €1.4 billion came as a shock to the politicians and the public.

Harris went out to bat on the project, somehow claiming the rise in costs was the result of a conscious decision by government to deliver a 'state-of-the-art' facility. Denying that spending was 'out of control', he said 'every single cent of this investment will be money spent on children's healthcare, and money that should have been spent decades ago'.

Few were buying these arguments, especially Harris's political opponents. 'It is unbelievable that in the space of two years the projected cost of delivering the national children's hospital has more than doubled from €650 million in 2016 to a projected €1.4 billion now,' said Labour health spokesman Alan Kelly in a press release. 'A 40 per cent increase in costs since spring 2017 cannot be brushed aside,' said Fianna Fáil health spokesman Stephen Donnelly.

Harris was feeling the political heat, as was his predecessor as minister for health Leo Varadkar, who was now taoiseach. Varadkar had been appointed to the top job in June 2017 at the age of 38, following Enda Kenny's resignation.

Living up to his reputation as a straight-talker, he declared that he was 'very concerned' at the rising cost of the hospital. 'We always expected that the price would rise as a result of construction inflation but the latest increase is way beyond what we had ever anticipated,' he said in December 2018 on a visit to the Blanchardstown urgent-care centre then under construction. It was clear the overrun would delay the delivery of other much-needed projects.

Harris attributed the increase to construction inflation and VAT for additional items. No fixed prices had been agreed for the main engineering and construction tenders for the project, he briefed cabinet, so subsequent reviews caused the price of tenders to increase.

The board started to feel the glare of public attention. 'No one defended us at that time,' says one member. 'No one backed the two-stage process, the one they are still using today.'

As the blame game widened, other ministers insisted their departments were 2not prepared to suffer for the budgeting failures in health. The government's room for manoeuvre was limited. Abandoning the project was not seen as a realistic option, given the years of delay and controversy.

Officials considered putting the second part of the contract out to tender, effectively switching from BAM to another contractor once the site works were completed. 'There was a moment when the question arose as to whether we would continue with BAM or not,' says Leo Varadkar. 'There had been informal approaches made to Sisk. And I heard they were willing to take over the project. But it wasn't really a runner because there was strong advice that it would have to go back to tender at that point.' This, it was estimated, would involve a further two-year delay and an estimated €305 million in extra costs.

Despite the problems that were emerging, the public was getting no proper explanation for the enormous cost overrun and how much worse things could get. 'Is this the worst of it, or could the sum climb even higher towards €2 billion?' I asked in an *Irish Times* article that month, not knowing that officials were already worrying that the figure might rise so high. 'We were told at the time the tendering process was "highly competitive",' my piece continued, 'and that the tenders were independently peer-reviewed by construction experts familiar with big projects. We were also told that the estimated cost included provision for inflation, VAT and contingencies –

though construction inflation has doubled approximately to 7 per cent since 2014. Given the improvement in the economy, this was hardly unforeseeable.'

The impact of the cost overrun was being felt throughout the health service, in every part of the country, I pointed out: 'Wondering why your local hospital has so many patients on trolleys? Blame the children's hospital for eating into the capital budget and delaying the provision of new beds.

'Wondering why the X-ray machine was broken on your last hospital visit, or why the ambulance was late bringing you there? Blame the children's hospital overrun for hoovering up the money that should have gone to funding badly needed replacements for clapped out equipment.'

Inflation had indeed played a part in pushing up costs, but there were other factors, potentially more embarrassing for the development board and the government. The original pricing of the project was based on preliminary drawings that lacked detail and had to be revised substantially, one source familiar with the process told me. Whose fault was that? Aside from the sprinkler issue, other reasons for the rising cost of the project included delays in the finalisation of the design, unanticipated extra costs of building on a brownfield site and increases in the amount of materials needed – all factors intrinsic to the design and execution of the project.

The guaranteed maximum price of €1.433 billion, which had been finally agreed by BAM and the development board in November 2018, was still awaiting government approval. This represented an increase of at least €400 million since the definitive business case of little over a year earlier.

Making savings was not an option, and neither was cancelling the project or finding a new contractor to build the hospital. Just before Christmas, the government bowed to the inevitable. 'A gun had been put to its head,' one former board member tells me. 'It had to agree to the increased price.'

Ministers approved the new budget, said to be the 'least-worst option' for delivering the hospital. Admitting this figure could rise further, Varadkar sought to make the best of a bad situation; the hospital might turn out to be the most expensive in the world, he told the Dáil, but it would be the best.

The project had been based on an agreed maximum price with the contractor, he explained, but within that there were 'elements' around tendering and cost inflation. In other words, though he didn't say it, the maximum price was not actually a maximum.

Along with design changes and new fire regulations, increased labour costs and a failure to make anticipated savings, the build was going to take nine months longer. Some €319 million was attributable to increased cost of construction, €50 million was due to VAT payments and the remainder was for a range of issues, including hospital equipment.

Still, with formal approval from cabinet, construction of the seven-storey building could finally begin in January 2019, following more than a year of below-ground works. The long-awaited hospital was now expected to be ready in August 2022, with the extra nine months of construction adding €90 million to the final bill.

The €1.43 billion figure for building the hospital wasn't the complete cost of the project. This came to €1.73 billion when other elements were included – building the urgent-care centres in

Tallaght and Blanchardstown, providing IT and electronic health record facilities, creating a new research centre, integrating the existing three children's hospitals and accounting for the money lost on the aborted earlier attempt to build the facility at the Mater.

A list was drawn up of other health projects that could be affected by the cost overruns at the children's hospital – promised extra hospital beds in Limerick, 90 care homes for older people, primary-care centres in three locations, a new emergency department and cystic fibrosis unit at Beaumont Hospital.

The original estimate for the project should have better reflected its scale and complexity 'relative to the capacity of the Irish construction market on a difficult congested site in a city-centre location', according to an internal memo, and a 'more robust' early-warning process should have been in place during the design phase. At this late stage, those behind the project were acknowledging difficulties with the site at St James's, saying that, by the time problems were noticed, it was too late to do anything about them.

'When all the bills are paid four or five years from now, the price of the state's biggest construction project will probably come close to €2 billion,' I predicted in December 2018. 'Throughout this period, there will be little money to build anything else in the health sector, unless the purse-strings are loosened further. The scale and complexity of the project appear to have been underestimated. As a consequence, earlier estimates of the cost involved were far too low.'

The Irish economy had continued to rebound strongly after the economic crash. Demand for badly needed infrastructure came roaring back, but many builders had gone out of business or left the country during the crisis. The project was proofed up to 4 per cent inflation, but with rates running well above this, BAM and the other main contractors were due bigger payments.

Spending on other major projects could be halted or curtailed for up to five years, Harris warned colleagues in a confidential cabinet memo in December 2018.

The projected cost of operating the hospital was also revised upwards, from an earlier estimate of €325 million a year to €366 million. Integrating the three existing children's hospitals would cost a further €86 million. 'We may end up building one of the most expensive children's hospitals in the world,' Varadkar mused at a pre-Christmas briefing with journalists. 'I can live with that if it turns out to be one of the best. But I don't want to have a children's hospital which is one of the most expensive to run.'

The taoiseach, who had been minister for health until a few years previously, expressed himself 'very dissatisfied' at the soaring cost of the hospital. This should have been anticipated, he said, given that it was being developed by a dedicated and experienced build board.

In an effort to raise funds privately to offset the overspend, officials at the Department of Health contacted naming rights specialists. Following the Phoenix hospital debacle, the planned facility had remained nameless, despite a grassroots campaign to have it named after Dr Kathleen Lynn, the 1916 volunteer and founder of the child-centred St Ultan's Hospital.

Harris told fellow ministers there was a very strong case to be made for getting naming rights sponsorship for parts of the hospital, and potential for selling the name of the hospital itself.

In the US, he pointed out, a children's hospital in Miami had changed its name after a $60 million (€51 million at the time) pledge by the charitable foundation of golfer Jack Nicklaus. Ohio's Nationwide Children's Hospital was rechristened after an insurance company of that name donated $50 million (€50 million).

The proposal to sell off the name of the hospital was quickly abandoned once it leaked, though Harris left open the possibility that areas within the building might be offered for naming sponsorship. 'The chopping and changing of names only serves to raise more hackles and is emblematic of a project that has lost both its identity and its way,' Professor Chris Fitzpatrick, former master of the Coombe, observed in an article in *The Irish Times*.

The decision left Ronald McDonald House – funded by the charitable arm of McDonald's – as the only commercial arrangement in place at the hospital. The fast-food chain's involvement in providing parent accommodation in a 52-bed block beside the new hospital, which followed on from a similar facility at Crumlin hospital, was criticised as inappropriate by the HSE's main anti-obesity expert. Professor Donal O'Shea described the positioning of the house at the entrance to the hospital as 'incredible' at a time of an obesity epidemic driven by ultra-processed foods.

The department again looked at options for 'descoping' (reducing) the project to save money, but found they offered 'very limited' savings of €79 million. Embarrassingly, this would leave it with fewer beds than were in the existing three children's hospitals.

And the new hospital was again aiming to raise €150 million a year through philanthropy, an ambitious target given the uncertainty and delay around the project and the bad press over runaway costs.

The arrival of Christmas saved the government from further scrutiny but it faced an inevitable barrage of criticism when the Dáil returned in January 2019. There was nothing for it but to draw the sting of the opposition attack by resorting to the time-honoured ploy of calling in outside consultants.

The HSE commissioned consulting firm PwC to conduct a review of the increase in costs and to identify potential weaknesses in the project, at an initially estimated cost of €450,000.

As the consultants began their work, the Oireachtas health committee and the Dáil public accounts committee opened separate hearings into the issue. 'In my political career, I have never seen a project so completely out of control in terms of cost,' veteran Labour leader Brendan Howlin declared. 'Even the expanded cost, which was originally €450 million but more realistically €650 million, is now likely to be three times that figure. How can that be?'

'A combination of ineptitude, lack of oversight and insouciance at the highest level of our public service means that an outrageously cavalier approach to taxpayers' money is being tolerated by the Government,' wrote financial commentator David McWilliams in

The Irish Times. 'It's not corruption, but it is a blatant failure of the process of public tendering.'

The scandal was wiping the sheen off two of the government's big names, Varadkar and Harris. As Harris wrestled with the mess, Varadkar sought to brush off opposition claims that he was a key contributor to it. While he was minister for health when planning permission was secured at St James's, he pointed out, that he had moved to the Department of Transport when the decision was made to build there and to Social Protection when the decision on tendering was made.

'I was a member of all of those governments. Therefore, I accept collective responsibility for the decisions in question,' he added. But not *personal* responsibility was the clear implication.

The development board appeared to have few regrets. 'If we were to start again on a project of this scale and complexity, we would adopt the same procurement approach,' its chairman, Tom Costello, told the committee. The board and its executive team had set about the task in a competent and professional manner, he said, using the most appropriate processes based on best international practice.

The tender process had attracted high-calibre bidders, and BAM had submitted a 'very competitive' tender. The two-stage procurement process had allowed initial construction work to begin two years earlier than if traditional methods had been employed: 'The process of determining the costs of the various packages was fully interrogated, independent reviews were commissioned.'

The hospital was a huge project and would result in one of the biggest children's hospitals in the world, Costello continued. However, it was also extraordinarily complex, and the infrastructure needed to deliver a fully digital hospital using electronic patient records was 'absolutely enormous'. The complexity of these services was not fully recognised in the early-stage design, Costello acknowledged.

Having examined other possibilities, including not going ahead with the contractor, 'the option of choosing BAM Ireland was by a large margin the best choice in terms of cost and certainty', the former chief executive of Sisk told the committee.

The facility was designed with more than 6,000 rooms, and this had had a cost impact, project director John Pollock pointed out. Each room would have multiple data points and, to protect against crashes, there was a need for a 'huge amount of duplication' including back-up systems, power supplies and generators.

Asked how many extra beds were being delivered for the additional €500 million being spent, he answered, 'There's no extra beds.'

While politically, the hospital had become a touchstone for controversy, on the ground relations remained civil. Earlier, the development board and its three main contractors had agreed to allow an additional five months for finalisation of the guaranteed maximum price. BAM had made additional claims and these had been settled without any great fuss.

In February 2019, a 'partnership seminar' for site workers was held in a west Dublin hotel. Those present discussed ways of improving systems and collaboration on-site. 'It went fantastically. People felt they had been treated fairly,' says a board source. 'BAM were tough, but we knew that was the way they behaved and you had to deal with it.'

16

Resignations, Reports and Recriminations

'The nation has been let down by those entrusted to manage its health service. The failure to have a final design before signing construction contracts is the fundamental flaw in this project.'

Dr Michael Harty, chair of the Oireachtas health committee and a GP from County Clare

'[We have] 5,000 km of cable, of all different sizes, and we have rates for each type of cable, but the actual quantum of it was not fully defined in the documentation.'

Project director John Pollock on the complexities of costing the project

Internal documents provided to the health committee and the public accounts committee in early 2019 shed light on how the overrun occurred, who knew about it and when they were told.

The two-stage procurement process had indeed allowed BAM to get on with clearing the site and creating the foundations. In this first stage, the contractor had provided a preliminary indication of the costs of constructing the seven-storey building. The detailed design specification for this featured only in the second phase of the tender.

There was a problem: although the prices of materials were nailed down at an early stage, the quantities were not. The bill of quantities submitted in the first phase of the tender for constructing the hospital was 'approximate and remeasurable'. It was not until the second phase that a full bill of quantities was provided.

Those designing the building underestimated the complexity involved – not just for construction but also for the mechanical and electrical services. 'At the early stage of the design, the complexity of those services and the quantities involved were not fully recognised within the early-stage tender. That became clear as the design developed over 2018,' Tom Costello explained at one committee hearing.

John Pollock instanced the use of electrical cable. '[We have] 5,000 km of cable, of all different sizes, and we have rates for each type of cable, but the actual quantum of it was not fully defined in the documentation.'

The complexity of the mechanical and electrical systems in particular – all 24 of them – was underestimated. With more than 6,000 rooms to equip, that resulted in a major under-calculation of costs.

'We were badly let down by the quantities being entirely incorrect,' Simon Harris told the Oireachtas health committee in February 2019. 'The cost of a widget is still at 2016 [prices], but they need a hell of a lot more widgets.'

Up to the middle of 2018, the project had been – officially at least – on budget, according to the monthly reports sent by the design team to the development board. But as mentioned earlier, Pollock had already drawn attention to issues with contractors in his meetings with department officials the previous March and April. In June 2018, he was more specific, referring to cost pressures, design gaps, delays and friction with contractors.

By August, the project team was signalling an estimated €191 million cost overrun. Officials warned that €200 million in additional cost claims were on the way from BAM and said there was still work to be done on calculating the overall size of the overrun.

In early September, Harris was told of 'grave concerns' about the extra costs. Yet later that month, in response to a Dáil question, he routinely answered that the project was within budget and cited a cost of €987 million.

With contract discussions with BAM nearing completion, Costello had asked officials to sign a confidentiality agreement so that 'no issues' leaked out. Different scenarios for controlling the bad news about the hospital overspend were war-gamed with the development board's public relations firm, Q4PR.

On 19 September, the programme board raised concerns that construction costs were 'trending very significantly over budget'. The enormous scale of the overrun had become apparent. Pollock went through the nuts and bolts of the cost creep – almost literally. There were changes to doors, materials, partitions and sockets, and mechanical and electrical items had been 'missed' in the bill of quantities.

On 9 November, Harris was told the project was €450 million over budget. At this point, the development board said the cost of constructing the hospital had risen to €1.43 billion.

The chronology appears to show that Harris was made aware in August 2018, two months before that year's budget, that cost overruns at the hospital could reach €400 million, when BAM's additional claims were included. But it wasn't until early November that the actual cost 'crystallised', the minister contends, thereby allowing political decisions to be made.

He says he had 'a sense' of the costs rising from the summer or autumn of 2018 but only got 'solid information' in November. 'Generally as a minister, you wait until information has been crystallised and clarified,' he tells me, 'rather than operating on a "Minister, we think there may be concerns or issues or further claims" basis. In August, my officials were telling me, "challenges here, problems, bit worried, BAM, new claims". Ultimately we updated the government once we had that clarity, in December.'

Harris also points to a 'back and forth' with the Department of Public Expenditure during this period: 'The Department of Health officials weren't just sitting there doing nothing. They were engaging with DPER [Department of Public Expenditure and Reform].' No time was lost and no extra cost incurred by waiting for the information to crystallise at the end of the year, rather than acting in August, he maintains.

Cost pressures were greater for the mechanical and electrical systems than for the construction element of the project, a briefing note from the Department of Health in January 2019 revealed. The share of the tender price due to BAM for building the hospital was €432 million in 2017 but grew to €556 million a year later, an increase of 29 per cent. Jones Group, which won the contract for the mechanical systems, originally tendered at €107 million, but this grew to €177 million, an increase of 65 per cent. The cost of the electrical systems contract won by Mercury Engineering rose from €98 million to €157 million, a 60 per cent rise.

The public had remained in the dark for years about the cost of the hospital. Back in February 2014, an internal estimate based on the work of quantity surveyors at the Mater put this at €800 million. Yet this figure was not made public and the quoted estimate remained at €650 million. It was only in 2017 that the board set a revised budget of €790 million, later €800 million.

A second issue reared its head during the investigations taking place: just who was in charge of the project?

The original idea had been simple: set up a board with the specific remit to build the new hospital and operate it. Leave behind the medical and local politics that bedevilled the project in its previous incarnations and populate the board with experts with lots of business and healthcare experience and a singular focus.

That was why the National Paediatric Hospital Development Board was established in 2007, its members appointed by the minister for health and its functions set out in legislation.

Then in 2013, following a decision by James Reilly, the job of merging the three existing hospitals and operating the new one was hived off to the Children's Hospital Group, later Children's

Health Ireland (CHI). The development board survived, but was repopulated with experts in construction, architecture and law.

In April 2017, further layers of governance and oversight were added, including a Children's Hospital Project and Programme Board chaired by the secretary-general of the Department of Health and a Children's Hospital Project and Programme Steering Group chaired by the deputy director general of the HSE.

Confused? The politicians certainly were. At the hearings of the health committee over several weeks in January 2019, members repeatedly asked the HSE and Department of Health witnesses why so many extra layers of governance had been put in place and who exactly was in charge.

Creating a 'build board' filled with like-minded people from construction backgrounds to build the hospital might have seemed a good idea on paper. It certainly ticked the boxes for expertise and focus. However, with just one project to take care of, the danger was that the board failed to tackle other important considerations.

It didn't have to worry about what other health projects were deserving of support or what other projects in other government departments should be advanced. Its job was to get the hospital built. Did this mean that cost considerations were always likely to be farther down the priority list?

As I wrote that February: 'Put together a flagship project, a Government desperate for an achievement to put down on its CV and a board more focused on building than cost management, and you have what some critics label "a licence to print money".'

Or, as a children's doctor put it to me: 'We got the colocation bit right. What we didn't get right was who was going to build this damn hospital.'

TDs identified as a clear flaw of the two-stage procurement process the difficulty of changing horses midstream, after BAM had been awarded the first phase of the contract. It was theoretically possible for the second phase to be awarded to a different contractor, but what other firm would want to arrive so late to a project, building on top of the foundations laid by one of their rivals? If something went wrong, who would be to blame?

As Fianna Fáil TD John Brassil told the health committee: 'The company that got phase one was also going to get phase two. It could do what it liked with the price, and it did so.'

BAM knew that it 'had it in the bag from day one. It knew that once it was on-site ... it was cushioned by the desperate need for a new children's hospital. It knew that we were stuck', Fine Gael TD Kate O'Connell told the same hearing.

BAM has consistently denied allegations of 'lowballing' made at this time and subsequently. It's worth remembering that the company's original tender, while lower than those of its competitors, came in higher than the board's own estimate of costs. And as noted previously, the cost of the electrical and mechanical tenders increased faster than its building tender. Underestimating of costs began long before BAM was involved with the children's hospital; the history of the project is full of oddly low estimates. In 2012, for instance, St James's, which stood to gain hugely in terms of prestige and size through the addition of a children's hospital to its adult facilities, estimated 'total construction costs' at a mere €297.75 million.

Before this, the development board wasn't given to complaining about its main contractor, certainly not in public. That was to change once the political pressure increased. And yet the booming economy was clearly impacting heavily on the project. General inflation in 2017 was a modest 0.36 per cent and wage inflation was 2 per cent, but construction tender inflation grew by 18–22 per cent between 2016 and 2018. A buoyant market, skills shortages and Brexit were said to be the driving factors.

Under ferocious political pressure from the evidence emerging from the committee meetings, Harris vowed at the start of February 2019 to make personnel changes. He also pledged accountability, although the PwC review was not empowered to assign individual liability. 'People will be held to account. There will be governance changes in relation to this, of that there is no doubt,' the minister promised.

Tom Costello announced his resignation the following day, saying concerns about reputational damage to the project from the costs controversy had forced his decision. He had lasted five years in the role.

From a previous dearth of information, the public arena was flooded with reports. Yet another set of consultants, Mazars, appointed by the development board to conduct an internal audit, found that a lack of early-warning systems had left the hospital board unable to lessen the €450 million increase in the project's cost. Its fundamental systems and checks and balances 'failed to protect the board from a large sudden increase in the cost of construction'.

The budgeting process 'failed to determine and therefore secure the necessary capital budget' from the beginning and 'failed to properly estimate the likely future costs of the project within the stated contingency limits'.

The stable door was being shut firmly now that the horse had bolted. Building the children's hospital at St James's rather than on a greenfield site in Dublin had added up to 5 per cent a year to the cost of construction, a separate report commissioned by the project board showed. It didn't sound too much, but over ten years that meant a cumulative increase of up to two-thirds in costs.

Another report by Linesight, the project's quantity surveyors, reviewed the cost of 15 hospital projects internationally and ranked the St James's project as the third most expensive.

'The nation has been let down by those entrusted to manage its health service,' the quietly spoken Dr Michael Harty, chairman of the health committee, concluded in February 2019. 'The failure to have a final design before signing construction contracts is the fundamental flaw in this project.'

With the government planning to splash out over €100 billion on Ireland's next national development plan, the overspending on the children's hospital stood out as a bad example. Would the mistakes made at St James's be repeated across the country as railways and roads, utilities and hospitals were built or renovated? Officials across the civil service scrambled to put in place controls designed to avoid a repeat.

~

The health committee had just concluded its investigation of overspending on the children's hospital, while the PwC report was imminent. It was hard to see how things could get any worse and yet they did.

It was early February 2019, and Leo Varadkar had been on his feet for over half an hour in the Dáil, defending his government's record on the hospital, given the colossal rise in costs.

The taoiseach accepted responsibility for the underestimation of costs and admitted that setting up a special development board to lead the project might not have been the right thing to do. He blamed construction inflation for some of the increase but insisted that the government had no alternative but to press on.

Nearing the end of leaders' questions, Varadkar made what seemed like a throwaway remark: 'We have a real concern that some companies have been lowballing, coming in with very low tender prices to get the contract and then coming back with claims thereafter. There are one or two contractors who, quite frankly, I would not like to see get a public contract again in this state.'

'Absolutely,' chimed opposition TD Richard Boyd Barrett.

'However, EU procurement law does not allow us to ban people from tendering,' Varadkar continued. 'Perhaps we can work into the scoring system a public service reference or a past form clause looking at previous projects.'

Up to this point, the blame for soaring costs at St James's had been fairly evenly distributed. True, government TDs had accused BAM of aggressively pursuing claims, but a failure to complete the design of the hospital before the contract was signed was also recognised as a major contributory factor to rising costs. Now, however, the taoiseach was squarely making accusations of lowballing contracts, and suggesting certain companies should be excluded from state contracts for engaging in it. No one was in any doubt about the firm he was referring to.

BAM Ireland chief executive Theo Cullinane quickly learned of the taoiseach's remarks. Cullinane, a tough-talking Corkman, was a BAM 'lifer' – his entire career had been spent at the company, including 13 of 43 years of service as chief executive.

'Theo was raging. This was personal – both for him and the company,' says an informed source. 'He felt his lads building the hospital were being unfairly maligned.'

On-site disagreements were nothing new for Cullinane and his crew at St James's. In the main, these were sorted out and understandings reached, according to both BAM and development board sources. Rows still happened, as on many building sites, but in most cases they were resolved between the parties. Where this wasn't possible, either side could go to arbitration.

The strains here had increased as cost expectations of the development board and its main contractor started to diverge. And now the taoiseach seemed to be directly blaming Cullinane's company for the problems at the children's hospital project, in a way that could threaten its public sector work more generally.

The Corkman wrote to Varadkar the following day, saying his 'inappropriate and damaging' remarks had been 'seriously damaging' to the company's reputation. He demanded the taoiseach immediately clarify that he was not referring to BAM in the Dáil and state that his company was 'in full compliance with all its obligations' at the children's hospital. He gave Varadkar a two-hour ultimatum to reply or else BAM would consider 'all our options'.

'The relationship with BAM was already very bad at that point,' says Varadkar, 'not just because of the children's hospital but also due to Grangegorman. I remember saying what I did and knowing that it was under Dáil privilege.'

The former taoiseach is unrepentant. 'BAM's letter demanding a correction/clarification cum apology within hours was no way for a contractor to behave towards a dissatisfied customer. It was further evidence of their aggressive approach at the time. I did not comply.'

Called upon to clarify the remarks, his spokesman claimed at the time that the taoiseach was not referencing any specific company.

The public row was a defining event in the history of the project, according to sources in BAM and the development board. Any remaining spirit of collaboration on the ground evaporated as government ministers fixed their sights on BAM as the alleged cause of the project's many problems, and the building contractor dug in its heels.

'I was amazed,' says one member of the development board. 'I thought they [the remarks] were totally inappropriate. BAM had been fair up to that point in time. The GMP [guaranteed maximum price] we arrived at should have been celebrated, but for whatever reason the board had no champion. Then everyone started covering their ass and finding someone to blame.' As he highlights, nobody was pointing the finger at the other contractors for the steep rise in their costs.

Left-wing TDs such as the builder turned independent TD for Wexford, Mick Wallace, were happy to continue the government's work by blaming – and naming – the contractor. 'If we continue with this procurement and this contract process, this project will not be built for €1.7 billion nor will it be built for an extra €500 million. I guarantee that the costs will not stop at €2.2 billion because this process is tailor-made for BAM to reef us,' he shouted from the floor of the Dáil the following day, before being shut up by the leas-cheann comhairle for naming an individual company. 'It will rob us blind with this form of an arrangement,' Wallace continued.

Yet the cost overrun would have materialised even if a contractor other than BAM had been selected to build the project, according to a HSE report into the price-setting process. Even though the company's bid was significantly lower than the next lowest, the same problem with price increases would have arisen with other bidders because of inflation and changes to the amount of materials needed for the project, it found.

Ultimately, Harris weathered the storm, while suffering significant political damage. In late February 2019, he narrowly survived a Sinn Féin motion of no-confidence, by 58 votes to 53. The minister had Brexit to thank for his survival; Fianna Fáil abstained in the vote because it did not want to risk an election with the UK's departure from the European Union looming in under a year's time.

'We will build the children's hospital after decades of debate, we will get to the bottom of what has gone wrong, we will ensure lessons are learned,' Harris vowed in his Dáil speech. 'But we will not walk away from this vital project.'

Attention focused on Paul Quinn, a senior official of the Department of Public Expenditure, the government's chief procurement officer and a member of the hospital development board. Why had he not raised concerns about the escalating cost externally, TDs on the health committee wanted to know.

'The chief procurement officer in the department was a member of the National Paediatric Hospital Development Board, yet he did not officially inform the department that there were serious concerns about unforeseen cost escalations, as it was not his board function to do so,' committee chairman Dr Michael Harty concluded.

Civil servants on state boards are obliged to pass on concerns to the relevant government minister if they feel these are not being dealt with and there is a public policy issue at stake, comptroller and auditor general Seamus McCarthy told the public accounts committee in February 2019.

In McCarthy's view, civil servants were bound by a circular stating that information should be presented to the minister where there were serious weaknesses in controls that had not been addressed, or where there was a risk of reputational damage to the body. As a non-commercial state body, the development board was subject to the rules of the circular.

But Paschal Donohoe said Quinn's responsibility was to the board itself. He was a member of a separate governance structure, the minister for finance explained.

'I would have been precluded and not only in breach of my obligations as a board member but also in breach of law if I were to report to the secretary-general or the minister,' Quinn told the public accounts committee in May 2019. Minister Donohoe had supported his stance when told of it, he added. Communications were taking place to ensure that the minister for health was 'absolutely apprised' of the issues.

After months in the eye of the storm, John Pollock tendered his resignation as project director in March 2019, shortly before the PwC report was due to be published. He had lasted five years and four months in the post.

His was the fifth prominent resignation from the benighted project – and it wouldn't be the last. Never one for the limelight, Pollock had appeared genuinely embarrassed by the cost overrun that occurred on his watch. The job had begun well, he noted, with a well-received design for the building and the securing of planning permission, before costs started spinning out of control. But then, I wrote at the time, he and the other members of the board were handed a poisoned chalice because the cost of building the hospital had been consistently underestimated in the early stages.

In April 2019, the long-awaited PwC report was published.

Described by Varadkar as 'grim reading', it told the public much of what it already knew, following the months of scrutiny of the project at Oireachtas committees.

Most of the €450 million overrun on the project since 2017 was down to an underestimation of the initial costs, the consultants' report suggested. There were 'significant failures' in planning and budgeting, and all but €16 million of the overrun could have been controlled.

'Red flags' around the inadequacy of the budget were missed from as early as the tendering stage in 2017. The report pointed to 'material errors' in the definitive business case on which the government made its decision to invest in the hospital at a cost of €983 million in April 2017. This overstated confidence in its forecasts and understated the complexity and risks involved.

There was little scope for saving money at this stage, according to the consultants. Retendering was ruled out, and a change of site was not considered in the report. PwC warned that it might cost a good deal more than the projected €1.73 billion to build and equip the hospital.

The report featured 'no real baddies', I wrote. 'No names are mentioned. The finger of blame is weakly pointed at times, then wrenched away in a fog of mitigation. As for the loss of hundreds of millions of euro of public money ... "it's complicated"'.

The report analysed the claims made by contractors to that point, which totalled €258 million. These had been settled in conciliation at €94.5 million.

Of these claims, BAM's portion came to €163 million, resulting in conciliation awards totalling about €60 million. The largest single award (€38.1 million) was for preliminaries for the 'increased value of work' involved in setting up and operating the site. There was no mention in the report of lowballing or aggressive claim-seeking by BAM, though this was by now the favoured explanation of government ministers when asked about cost increases at the hospital.

The PwC report identified a series of problems in the planning and execution of the project, and described the original budget as 'flawed'. 'In defence of the board, it was too thinly resourced in the early stages,' says John Martin, a member for six years. 'We didn't have the executive staff needed to carry out all the functions of such a complex project. We had accountants but no planners or architects. Too much reliance was placed on the board members and whatever expertise and time they could bring to it.'

With government deciding to press ahead with construction, Harris and Paschal Donohoe were sent off to draw up measures aimed at strengthening project governance and putting in place more robust control systems.

'It was clear we were going to be in for a very significant period of claim and counter-claim,' Harris says. 'Senior government officials were urging us to keep the pressure on BAM, and to contact Royal BAM. We had a company that had bid at a certain price, but was going to fight for every claim. Then we got dogged, and we are to this day.'

High in the sky above Dublin 8, a drone could be seen flying once a week over the construction site of the hospital during 2019, an indication of the breakdown in trust between the development board and BAM. Unhappy with the level of information flowing from the contractor, the board had engaged a UK firm of forensic project managers to monitor progress from the sky.

'They [BAM] were tough negotiators,' says a source who helped lead the project during this period. 'There was no willingness to resolve issues. They'd fight their case very hard. They were experts at itemising everything.'

There has to be give and take in every big project, as costs fluctuate according to the design challenges encountered along the way. In many projects, gain-sharing arrangements operate between the client and the contractor, whereby savings made are shared between both parties. 'BAM paid lip-service to gain-sharing, but they weren't really committed to it,' says the source. 'It turned into a dogfight over everything.'

This he ascribes to a 'corporate attitude' on the part of the contractor, though relations between managers on the site were also poor. 'There was no willingness to resolve issues.'

'Relations between the board and BAM seemed to be permanently fractious,' says Paul Reid, who was appointed chief executive of the HSE in May 2019, just after the PwC report was published. 'There was some scurrying around to put in the right structures, and to fill the gaps that were there. I found the governance structures for the project confusing. It was hard to see who was in charge. Although I wrote the cheques, I certainly never felt that I was in charge – and I wasn't. That seemed to fall to the development board, overseen by the Department of Health.

'I had enough to do,' Reid says. 'I wasn't particularly looking for it [control of the project]. It was a relief that something else was in place.'

The development board, funded from the public purse but

operating in the private sector, had its own challenges. 'The private sector attitude was "get the job done", while the public sector's was "go cheap and look over your shoulder"', a source tells me. 'They wanted the cheapest, and I wanted what worked.'

This manager relied on contractors to plug staffing gaps, because the salaries on offer were too low for a project of this size. The lack of bonuses – common in the private sector – was also a hindrance. 'Sometimes, I'd recruit someone or buy software and not tell the HSE beforehand; otherwise it wouldn't happen.' Project managers working on private-sector jobs as big as the children's hospital could expect to earn up to €1 million a year, including performance pay, he points out.

Still more delays ensued. The site was congested, there were restrictions on night work and it was proving difficult to source workers – and a replacement for Pollock. In June 2019, construction work was halted for two weeks because of 'wind exposure'.

More development board members resigned, including Paul Quinn. BAM submitted more claims for extra fees and extensions of time. 'There will always be rows in construction over cost and time; it's in the nature of the industry. I would say the main contractor on the job, BAM, is probably a little more active in this regard than many other contractors are,' new development board chairman Fred Barry told TDs in June 2019.

Barry had been appointed the previous February to fill the gap left by Tom Costello's departure and took up the post in April. As a former chief executive of the National Roads Authority, Barry had long experience of working with BAM on the construction of motorways, which was presumably why he was appointed.

The urgent-care centre in Blanchardstown opened at the end of July after a relatively painless build, though its operating hours were restricted initially over staffing issues. In the first month, attendances ran at under half the expected levels. The other urgent-care centre, in Tallaght, was delayed. It was forecast to open in 2020, with the new children's hospital now due to open in 2023.

In September 2019, the development board recorded its fifth resignation of that year, when paediatrician Jonathan Hourihane, the only doctor on the board, stepped down.

'I joined that board as the representative of the Faculty of Paediatrics, thinking it was for the development of services and planning [for the running of the new hospital] but that was the other board [CHI],' he tells me. 'The development board was talking about pipes, road closures, truck deliveries, contracts. I couldn't understand why a faculty rep had been put there. When it came to the point where they were trying to reappoint the group with chairman number two or three, I said, "Listen, I don't think you need me. I'm getting nothing out of this." So I resigned, and that faculty representation stopped. I was a witness more than a participant.'

To deal with the worsening situation, the government called in the cavalry – or, at least, a former army officer. In September, David Gunning was appointed to the newly created post of chief officer of the development board, effectively tasked with completing the long-delayed hospital. An engineer by profession and a former chief executive of Coillte, Gunning started his career in the Defence Forces, serving for ten years in the communications and information services corps. Other than telecoms masts, he had no construction experience. His record in health was limited to a stint as chief executive of Royal Hospital Donnybrook, a small and long-established rehabilitation facility in south Dublin.

Gunning was 'no shrinking violet', a former senior civil servant tells me. 'He was built for an adversarial environment.'

'David didn't have prior experience at that level, but he could handle himself,' says a staffer in the development board. 'He was head and shoulders above everyone else.'

That same month, Dublin City Council slapped a one-week ban on out-of-hours construction after permitted working hours at St James's were breached. Acting on residents' complaints, the council found that on some days construction began at 6 a.m. and continued almost until midnight. The pouring of concrete and other works continued on Saturday and Sunday. Vibration levels exceeded limits on a handful of days over the summer.

The residents who had gone to court in 2017 restarted their legal action, claiming there had been 'movement' to their houses.

By the end of 2019, the government was in deep trouble, principally on the issues of housing and health. In December, minister for housing Eoghan Murphy survived a motion of no-confidence by just three votes. Defeat would have forced Varadkar to call a general election.

In the event, he did just that a month later. Rural independents tabled another motion of no-confidence in Harris, alleging mismanagement of the children's hospital project and other health initiatives. When a Fianna Fáil TD threatened to support the motion rather than abstain, and a normally supportive independent TD said he would abstain, the game was up. The government didn't have the numbers to win the vote and a general election was called for February 2020.

Strictly speaking, the children's hospital hadn't brought down the government, but it had shortened its life. Its impact was clear in the results of the election, in which Fine Gael lost 15 seats. And matters were about to get much, much worse.

17

Plague Hospital

'It's been dogged in secrecy along the way. It is a defining illustration of this government's hands-off approach to major projects. They are more interested in the photo ops than they were in getting it done on time.'

Fianna Fáil leader Micheál Martin, in opposition in 2020, complaining about the government's approach to the children's hospital

'I have no intention of giving a ballpark figure because it would disadvantage the taxpayer and the state to announce to the contractor the level at which you want to go to.'

Micheál Martin, speaking as taoiseach, November 2022

By the start of 2020, construction of the children's hospital and its foundations had been underway for more than three and a half years. Relations between the development board and its main contractor, BAM, had deteriorated further. Delays were a constant, with rising costs the backdrop to ever-sharper rows.

The previous October, BAM had presented a new programme containing revised construction timelines, but the board claimed these were 'not in line with what is in the contract'. It blamed 'an exceptional level of claims' by the contractor. The board needed €15 million to defend itself against these claims, it told the HSE and government officials.

BAM questioned the validity of the board's earlier instruction to proceed with the second phase of work. This should not have happened, the contractor maintained, because the design was not ready. This was to crystallise as a core point of dispute, with BAM claiming it was instructed to start building a massive structure in January 2019 without a complete design in place, and the development board insisting that the instruction was fully valid.

Delays of 131 days for the complex façade of the main hospital building and 58 days for the structural frame were notified to officials. Both would have cost implications down the line.

Small wonder that then minister for finance Paschal Donohoe, when asked in January 2020 what his biggest regret was in politics, answered: 'not managing the national children's hospital better ... I will always look back at the controversy ... and challenge myself as to how I could have done that better'.

With the project now a touchstone for controversy, every aspect attracted media attention. Concerns around surveillance and possible espionage were expressed in relation to the hospital's plans to use facial recognition CCTV bought from a company backed by the Chinese state. Separately, Eilish Hardiman warned that one of the biggest challenges for the hospital when it opened would be finding the 1,600 nurses needed to staff it. The hospital was looking at possible NHS-style apartment developments for staff along connecting Luas and bus lines, she suggested. This idea wasn't heard of again.

Though years behind schedule and way off budget, the project had now at least settled into something of a rhythm. Despite all the fractiousness and finger-pointing, construction was proceeding steadily and an impressive building was taking shape on the western end of the St James's campus.

But even this fragile progress was to be shattered as that spring arrived. The year had opened with brief reports of a mystery virus originating in China, but within weeks Covid-19 was sweeping across the world. The new virus spread from country to country like wildfire, forcing bewildered governments to introduce swingeing restrictions on ordinary life.

Ireland, which reported its first case on 29 February, was no different. A fortnight later, Varadkar (still taoiseach while haggling over the formation of the new government continued) announced the closure of schools in an effort to stem the spread of the virus. By the end of March, the health service was deluged with cases, dozens of people had died and the government had announced a national stay-at-home order.

Here was the black-swan event some critics had warned of, a rare occurrence that was extremely difficult to predict but was always more likely to occur the longer a megaproject like the children's hospital dragged on. By any number of previous timelines – all long since ripped up – the hospital should have been built by this time. But it wasn't, and so Ireland's biggest construction project was facing a total shutdown.

At first, BAM kept the site open. The company referred to a government announcement that exempted some large-scale construction projects from restrictions and said it was seeking clarity from the development board. In the absence of a declaration that the hospital project was not an 'essential' construction project, work continued.

An opposition TD accused the contractor of putting lives at risk by 'demanding' that staff continue to work. BAM pointed out that its motorway-maintenance division was exempt from the shutdown edict, and said it was awaiting guidance.

In reality, neither BAM Ireland nor the board wanted to take responsibility for closing the site, given that additional costs would accrue. Talks were followed by a statement from the company saying the board had deemed the construction site non-essential. In its statement, the board ascribed responsibility for health and safety on the site to the company. It said BAM's 'obligation' was to shut down the site.

The next day, 31 March, work stopped.

By halting construction at St James's, the pandemic exacerbated tensions between the development board and its main contractor. BAM was left feeling it had been unfairly treated by the decision to deem the project non-essential. The closure of the country's largest construction site at the point of peak activity could lead only to more cost and delays.

Separately, the two sides' wider disputes, having exhausted internal conciliation mechanisms, moved to the High Court. In April 2020, the board began legal proceedings against BAM, seeking resolution of the differences over the validity of its instruction to start phase B works in January 2019. The case was sent for fast-tracking in the commercial court.

The row hinged on a claim by BAM that the board was required, under the contract signed in August 2017, to provide it with a 'complete fully coordinated' design before the phase B instruction was issued. The company claimed this was not provided as stipulated in the contract and the design remained incomplete.

As the government and the health service wrestled with the pandemic, and construction activity fell to its lowest level since the economic crash 11 years earlier, the future of the children's hospital was wreathed in uncertainty. There was speculation, later discounted, that the hospital could be delayed by three to four years due to the physical distancing measures under lockdown. In reality, no one knew at this point what was going to happen.

The lockdown became a new front in the war between BAM and the development board. Industry-wide restrictions were lifted on 18 May as the first wave of Covid-19 infections eased, but almost two months later work had yet to resume at the hospital site. Who should bear the cost of the closure and restricted reopening of the site? Social distancing measures in place had major cost implications for the relatively tight site at St James's, the cost of which BAM wanted met.

The company cried foul when it was excluded from a Covid-19-related compensation scheme for the construction sector, seemingly on the basis that the hospital was being built using a different contract from the standard public-works contract. Continuing pandemic restrictions would force it to halve the 2,000 workers needed on-site, it said in July.

As the site remained closed, the board pondered terminating its contract with BAM, until an exasperated new taoiseach, Micheál Martin, intervened that month. 'Why is it the children's hospital site [is] one of the few if only sites where work hasn't recommenced,' he asked. 'Work has recommenced on construction sites all across the country. People have gone back to building. It's unacceptable in my view what's happened here.' The builders should 'get back on-site and start building the children's hospital because the children of this country need it'.

The board issued the company with an indicative timeline for a return to work, and threatened legal action if it was not followed.

BAM agreed to resume operations 'in good faith' and 'in the interest of completing the project as quickly and economically as possible'. After a break of 14 weeks, the project was up and running again. Workers worked in bubbles of six and were tested for the virus twice a week.

Pandemic or no, the bills kept rolling in – €168 million was paid out to BAM out of a total spend of €469 million to the end of 2019. The overall sum included €1 million for Q4PR, the board's public-relations firm, for communications and community engagement work, and over €500,000 to lawyers McCann FitzGerald, much of it used in disputes with BAM.

As a letter-writer to *The Irish Times* put it: 'Our National Children's Hospital – the gift that keeps on taking.'

In opposition, Micheál Martin had claimed the children's hospital project was 'dogged in secrecy'. But now its affairs became even more opaque, with the board declining to estimate the ultimate cost or specify a completion date. Officials said they were precluded by non-disclosure agreements from discussing the costs of the hospital.

The officially cited cost remained €1.433 billion, with a further €300 million for fit-out, but this did not factor in inflation and the mounting number of claims being made by BAM, which were the subject of independent arbitration.

By November 2020, BAM had submitted more than 600 claims for extra costs, amounting to more than €200 million. Only a handful had been resolved.

The dispute between the board and its contractors settled into an established pattern, with board officials making accusations against BAM in their regular appearances before Oireachtas committees, and the company responding, often within hours, by way of statement from its public-relations advisors.

In November 2020, for example, development board chief officer David Gunning claimed at the health committee that the delays were down to BAM not providing sufficient resources for the project. He told TDs that BAM 'has been underperforming as regards project execution and has been extremely assertive as regards claims.'

BAM responded by statement, arguing that it had 'not received a fully complete, coordinated design for the project' and claiming new amendments were being added to the design 'all the time'. Almost 10,000 new drawings had been submitted since January 2019, it said: 'Therefore it is hardly surprising that there are hundreds of notifications from BAM and its major subcontractors of potential additional costs/delays.'

And yet Gunning had claimed the design upon which the tender was based was 'pretty complete and was accepted as so. We'd argue there hasn't been any significant change in terms of the scope of the project, what we're expecting to build'. Given the lack of transparency, it was difficult for an outsider to determine where right belonged in this dispute.

Nationally, further lockdowns followed as Covid-19 cases surged in a second wave in autumn 2020 but, this time, the building site was allowed to remain open. The hospital was ten months behind the timeline set down when BAM started construction, and another nine months would be needed to commission the hospital before it could receive patients. BAM's claims now numbered 700, with a combined value of €300 million.

Talk of hundreds of claims garnered attention but in reality most individual claims were minor enough – variations such as moving a door in a room, for instance – rather than large changes requiring conciliation, arbitration, planning amendments or legal remedies. A small number accounted for the bulk of the sums being claimed. BAM also complained of repetition, saying the contractual provisions resulted in 'replicating the same notification across a number of different areas or in successive months, although it is in essence the same notification'.

The war of words continued. Gunning, on yet another outing at the Dáil public accounts committee, accused BAM of underperforming and under-resourcing. 'This is a situation that has been in place since the beginning and which continues today,' he told the politicians. The board started withholding 15 per cent of monthly payments to the contractor until it was provided with a programme of works it regarded as compliant with the contract.

BAM, for the umpteenth time, rejected these accusations and claimed the main driver of delays and claims 'has been and continues to be the lack of a fully complete, coordinated design for the project.'

'These amendments result in, for example, requirements for additional materials, changes to quantities and specifications on materials, changes to entire work programmes on-site and scheduling of teams of subcontractors.'

By June 2021, the completion date had slipped to December 2023, and the opening day was forecast for the second half of 2024. BAM now had 900 outstanding claims – as defined by the board – but only nine had been settled at arbitration. Six of the bigger ones were in dispute and heading to the High Court.

Officially, the cost of building the hospital remained at €1.433 billion, not that anyone set any store in this figure. Gunning said it didn't include a number of items since 'there was no price certainty for them'. As provided for in the contract, BAM had begun receiving payments for the cost of construction inflation in excess of 4 per cent; these payments would obviously increase if inflation continued to rise. But wider statutory changes, or changes in healthcare policy, could influence the scope and, therefore, the cost of the project.

In the courts, it was the turn of BAM to sue the development board after mediation failed to resolve their differences over extra payments. These extra costs were allegedly the result of delays caused by incomplete design and incomplete design information.

Ciarán Fahy, a part-time conciliator appointed under the contract's dispute resolution mechanism, had made an award of €20 million to BAM, about 45 per cent of the amount originally sought, but this had been rejected by the board.

Department of Health officials, called before the public accounts committee in July, declined to provide an updated cost for the project. With a live commercial contract in place, it would be 'inappropriate and very likely detrimental' to speculate on the ongoing costs, Fiona Prendergast told TDs. Gunning too said he was not in a position to give a costs update but added that he was 'content' about the way claims were being defended.

When it was put to him that the project was likely to cost more than €2 billion, he said he would not commit to a ballpark final figure.

Seven months after they had started looking for figures, committee members were left to rail against a lack of transparency around the project. 'Nothing short of disgraceful,' said Fine Gael senator Martin Conway.

The committee reconvened the following week, and officials again refused to provide estimates of the final cost. To do so would compromise the board's ability to negotiate on behalf of the state, Gunning argued.

When she was asked about the €2 billion-plus estimate,

Prendergast replied that she was not prepared to discuss such a figure, adding, 'At no stage has this department ever considered a figure of €2 billion.'

In November 2021, the urgent-care unit in Tallaght opened with a promise by doctors that within three years there would be 'almost no waiting lists' for general paediatric care. At the time, more than 3,000 children were waiting to be seen by a consultant.

As the year came to a close, questions around the overall cost of the national children's hospital went further up the chain of command, though they remained unanswered. Department of Health secretary-general Robert Watt said any potential future costs outside the approved budget were commercially sensitive and had to remain confidential. Minister for public expenditure Michael McGrath said a final estimate was 'some distance off'.

'My very clear view is that publishing commercially sensitive information at this stage in a contract which is subject to dispute will be very damaging for state interests,' Watt told a heated meeting of the public accounts committee in December.

A moratorium on dealing with claims had been put in place in summer 2021 in order to prioritise the building of the hospital. Still, the number of claims made by BAM continued to mount, along with their cumulative value: disclosed as 1,023 in number, with a value of €554 million, in February 2022.

~

On 24 February 2022, Russia invaded Ukraine. The largest and deadliest conflict in Europe since the Second World War triggered a global energy and food crisis, the mass movement of refugees and disrupted supply chains. In Ireland, electricity and gas prices soared, inflation hit the highest level in 40 years and over 110,000 refugees arrived in the country.

Following on from the pandemic, here was another external event affecting the children's hospital, forcing up the prices of materials and labour and placing existing agreements under pressure – as if they weren't already.

Though most of the steel and concrete required had been installed at the site, the growing cost of energy, fuel and transport hit hard. Offcials forecast in June 2022 that hyperinflation in construction would add €51 million to overall costs over a four-year period. At this point, the building was said to be 70 per cent complete and had just been 'topped out' at the seventh floor.

Government strategy now boiled down to one aim: *Build the bloody thing*. The moratorium on claims had been put in place to kick differences between the board and its builder down the road. Officials' reluctance to cite cost figures was designed to avert further damaging headlines. The minutes of board meetings were posted online tardily and with ever-increasing redactions.

In October 2022, I asked the board why the minutes of any of its meetings that year were not online. A spokeswoman replied saying this was an 'oversight'. Shortly after, the minutes of meetings up to the previous April were placed on its website.

As usual, details relating to costs were redacted. The minutes did shed light on other problems arising during construction, such as the installation and of 'non-compliant [insulation] board' in an area of the new hospital, which was later replaced.

When Taoiseach Micheál Martin was given a tour of the site in November 2022, the media were asked along.

The interior of the building was taking shape. 'The hospital is still a hard-hat zone dominated by the buzz of machinery, but the elements of a sophisticated twenty-first-century healthcare facility are steadily beginning to emerge,' I wrote. 'It is hard not to be impressed by the level of design and thought applied to this project.

'The entrance is a vast concourse with wraparound stairs and the shafts where six panoramic lifts will be installed to take visitors to one of 4,800 clinical rooms ... There are cafes, an "all-faith facility" and a 350-seat auditorium where many of the 2,500 students will be trained. But the heart of the hospital are the 380 inpatient rooms for sick children, each one single-occupancy, wheelchair-accessible and en-suite.

'All of the cubicles enjoy natural light and a view, either onto the interior courtyard gardens or outward towards the Dublin mountains, the Phoenix Park or the city centre. The rooms were designed in consultation with child patients, whose wish list included a bed for parents staying over, mirrors and a full-size television for family movie-watching. There is air-conditioning, but the windows open. Each room will be equipped with a "child edutainment system", a handheld tablet which the young patient can use for education or amusement.'

The elevated helipad, the first of its kind in an Irish hospital, was expected to receive about four flights a week, each one landing on a roof expensively reinforced with hundreds of tons of steel. We were shown 22 rooms that would serve as operating theatres, located off a exceedingly long corridor – more than the 15 in the existing three Dublin children's hospitals.

Martin planted a tree on the grounds of the hospital and acknowledged the 'very difficult journey' the project had taken to get to this stage. Lessons had to be learned from the experience about the management of big projects, but what was important now was to 'keep the head down' and 'get completion'.

Back in the Dáil, he stuck to the same line adopted by his officials. 'I have no intention of giving a ballpark figure because it would disadvantage the taxpayer and the state' to announce to the contractor 'the level at which you want to go to', he told Sinn Féin leader Mary Lou McDonald. Never mind that, for the most part, the differences between BAM and the board would be decided in mediation or the courts.

'This whole saga has been an exercise of kicking the can down the road and God only knows where this will end up,' McDonald retorted.

Still, senior civil servants realised a day of reckoning was approaching. The new oversight group in the Department of Health told the development board and the HSE the final costs would have to be 'bottomed out', or stabilised.

With the existing budget all but spent, government approval was required for further funding. Meanwhile, it emerged that the electronic record system to be used in the children's hospital would not be compatible with different systems in use in many hospitals, including Crumlin, Temple Street and St James's. Worse, the cost of implementing Epic, likely to be the most complex healthcare IT system in the world, spiralled to €362 million, from an earlier estimate of €86 million.

The year 2023 brought little change to the established pattern of delays and stonewalling. The projected opening date of the hospital slipped back further as politicians and officials continued to dodge the cost question.

Fianna Fáil's Stephen Donnelly, minister for health since June 2020, said there was 'no agreed figure' for the final cost of the children's hospital. Declining to provide an estimate, he explained he didn't want to prejudice negotiations between the contractor and the board.

In May, it emerged that technical experts had flagged issues with the air-ventilation system fitted in the ceilings of half the hospital's operating theatres. The consultants warned that the issues identified were 'indicative of major generic faults' and the longer they took to get resolved, the more expensive and time-consuming they would be.

The problem could add 12 months and over €50 million to the project, Sinn Féin's health spokesman David Cullinane claimed on RTÉ Radio, based on his conversations with an unidentified whistleblower.

Officials downplayed the seriousness of the issue and said it remained to be seen who would pay for any remediation if needed. 'The change, if instructed to BAM, will involve the movement of four ceiling grilles in each of the 11 theatres,' according to a board statement in June 2023. 'This will not cost "tens of millions of euro", as is being claimed, and is not expected to have an impact on the completion date of the hospital.'

Once again, diametrically opposing versions of the same issue were being broadcast, leaving the public confused. The row generated more heat than light before BAM was sent back to work on the theatres. Ultimately, the problem was fixed by substituting circular grilles for square ones in 11 theatres. The board said this work cost €200,000, not the millions of euro Cullinane had suggested.

As the delivery date of the hospital slipped by another two months, board officials kept up their criticism of BAM, alleging low productivity and under-resourcing. Only 27 rooms at the hospital had been completed.

In July, Varadkar acknowledged the budget of €1.43 billion would have to be increased and that the original cost of the hospital had been 'substantially underestimated'.

Sinn Féin finance spokesman Pearse Doherty, richly mixing his metaphors, said the project had become a 'runaway train' and claimed that Stephen Donnelly was 'asleep at the wheel'.

The building was now 21 months behind schedule.

Donnelly, who in opposition had harried ministers about the cost of the hospital, adopted the line that 'nobody right now knows' the final bill. To specify an amount would open the state to further claims, he said.

The two sides found new things to argue over. The board engaged a leading international investigative and intelligence company to review works on the site. Founded in the 1970s by a US private detective, Kroll had tracked down the millions former president Ferdinand Marcos had stolen from the Philippines and Saddam Hussein's siphoned-off oil money in Iraq. The US corporate intelligence firm was also hired by film producer Harvey Weinstein when he was accused of sexual assault.

Kroll's investigators were shut out of the site for six weeks and BAM refused to attend meetings with them, according to the board minutes. Tasked with estimating a realistic completion date, Kroll formed the view that the contractor's timeline was optimistic. Further delays were likely.

The row rumbled on, with BAM saying 'the level of persistent change' to the hospital's design was responsible for variations that prompted additional claims, and the development board insisting that 'it is project delivery and not design that is impacting on the substantial completion date'.

Documents given to Sinn Féin provided an insight into the problems that were arising. More than 300 doors in the hospital were found not to meet 'the effective clear width and might have to be replaced or demolished'.

Relations between the board and BAM were at 'an all-time low', David Cullinane claimed. 'The board are alleging that the contractor is not deploying sufficient resources to complete the project. BAM are saying that they have been given thousands of design changes and all of this is delaying the project. And while this is happening, we know the cabinet will be signing off on hundreds of millions more of taxpayers' money.'

As the number of BAM's claims exceeded 2,000, Donnelly

appointed an expert in the resolution of contentious construction disputes, lawyer Susan Bryson, to the development board in August 2023.

The minister blamed the latest delays on three factors – the Covid-19 pandemic, the war in Ukraine and the necessity to fight BAM's claims, which now totalled an extra €760 million. The hospital was 90 per cent complete, he said.

At St James's, the slippage continued. With BAM said to be hitting only 65–66 per cent of its monthly performance targets, Varadkar acknowledged the opening date could 'slip again'.

Gunning reported improved conditions on the site, but the number of BAM's claims rose further, to almost 2,400.

In October 2023, the board announced the date for 'substantial completion' of the hospital as 29 October 2024, more than two years after the initially contracted date of August 2022. Fitting out and commissioning would take another six months at least. The prospect of children actually using the hospital before the next general election had faded.

18

The Trouble with Megaprojects

'... over budget, over time, under benefits, over and over again.'

Professor Bent Flyvbjerg's 'iron law of megaprojects'

'If people knew the real cost from the start,
nothing would ever be approved.'

Former San Francisco mayor Willie Brown on the merits of lowballing civic projects

As many a homeowner has learned, even the smallest house extension can run over budget and take longer than expected to complete. These challenges are greatly amplified in huge and complex construction projects such as Ireland's national children's hospital.

The world is littered with examples of megaprojects that have gone seriously wrong. Berlin's new airport cost three times the original estimate and opened nine years late. The Channel Tunnel cost more than twice the original forecast. Boston's Big Dig, a motorway project, came in more than 400 per cent over budget and nine years behind schedule. HS2, an ongoing high-speed rail project linking British cities, has doubled in cost, even though the original proposal has been scaled back, and it's likely to open at least 11 years late. The Sagrada Família cathedral in Barcelona is still being worked on, over 140 years after construction started (although, in this case, that may be the point).

Hospitals, one of the most complex types of modern building, are not immune to this pattern. The Royal Adelaide Hospital in Australia ran hundreds of millions of dollars over budget and was delayed for more than 18 months by legal disputes and design flaws. The same city is currently building a new women's and children's hospital, due for completion in 2031, that is expected to cost twice the original estimate. Closer to home, a new critical-care centre at Belfast's Royal Victoria Hospital was completed eight years late and 60 per cent over budget.

The national children's hospital is Ireland's megaproject, the biggest and most costly building ever constructed in the Republic. It is not a complete surprise, therefore, that it has shared the same fate as the examples I have just cited. And yet it is hard to understand how nothing was learned from the problems of other megaprojects to avert some of the issues that arose at the St James's site.

Overspending and missed deadlines are not givens in big projects. The Empire State Building in New York famously came in 17 per cent under budget and was built in just over a year. The world's highest building, the Burj Khalifa in Dubai, opened in 2010 on budget and only slightly late. In industry, Boeing took 28 months to design and build the first of its 747 planes. Less than a year elapsed between the time Apple hired the first employee to work on the iPod and shipping of the first product.

Professor Bent Flyvbjerg is the world's leading authority on the better management of megaprojects. You could say his life's megaproject is megaprojects. He maintains a database of these behemoths, extending to over 28,000 examples, from which he tries to learn lessons.

The wisdom of big numbers provides revealing insights. Nine out of ten megaprojects experience cost overruns, and just 0.5 per cent come in on budget and on time, while delivering the benefits promised. The mean cost overrun of hospital projects is 29 per cent – a lot lower than the overspend at St James's.

This analysis led Flyvbjerg to formulate his 'iron law' of megaprojects: they tend to run 'over budget, over time, under benefits, over and over again'. This, he argues, is not a random occurrence but the result of systemic, predictable failure.

Psychology and power play prominent roles in any big project, he points out, as people and organisations compete for resources and jockey for position. As for the causes of failure, he identifies two human biases that can drive plans awry.

The first is optimism bias, our tendency to underestimate risk and be overly disposed to looking on the bright side. This leads to fanciful estimates for costs, timetables and expected benefits of a project. Unless checked, optimism leads to unrealistic forecasts and poorly defined goals, he says in his book *How Big Things Get Done*, written with Canadian journalist Dan Gardner. Better options are missed and no contingency is made to counteract surprises.

Then there is what Flyvbjerg calls 'strategic misrepresentation', where the costs of a project are deliberately underestimated, and its benefits deliberately overestimated, to win funding and political approval. This can result in 'shallow analysis', followed by a 'quick lock-in' to a decision that sweeps aside all other options. People behave as if they have to push on, and end up accepting more costs or risks than they envisaged at the start.

This approach was best summed up by San Francisco's former mayor Willie Brown, who has argued with remarkable honesty that no one should be shocked by overruns on big projects with lowballed estimates. With public projects, the first budget is just a 'down payment', Brown wrote in a column in the *San Francisco Chronicle* in 2013. 'If people knew the real cost from the start, nothing would ever be approved. The idea is to get going. Start digging a hole and make it so big, there's no alternative to coming up with the money to fill it in.'

Another leading writer on megaprojects, Italian Riccardo Cosentino, has drawn parallels with, of all things, kitesurfing.

With kitesurfing, he writes, you have to assess whether you're dealing with normal wind or storm-driven wind. One carries the person smoothly, while the other 'can drag you into a situation you can't escape from'. With megaprojects and kitesurfing, heading into the unknown unprepared 'invites failure'. Success, in contrast, comes from 'equipping yourself with expert knowledge and the right tools'. And in both activities, holding on too long only makes a bad situation worse.

Flyvbjerg is not optimistic about curing the problems of

megaprojects but he does suggest a 'think slow, act fast' approach: meticulous, data-driven planning should be followed by high-speed execution of the project.

The lengthy duration of megaprojects makes it more likely that something unexpected – such as an election upset, a stock market collapse, a war or a pandemic – will derail them. Professor Flyvbjerg's proposal for minimising this possibility is to speed up execution and bring the project to a conclusion faster.

He also advocates a modular or 'Lego principle' in which giant projects are constructed simply from smaller, repeatable components. The Empire State Building, he points out, is just the same storey constructed again and again, on top of each other. Neither of these approaches was adopted at the children's hospital at St James's.

People don't expect big projects to be grand cultural landmarks or to be wildly creative and unusual, he says. But they do want them to be excellent, to finish on time and on budget and 'to do what they're supposed to do'.

'You can't always anticipate what's going to happen when you're building,' Irish barrister and construction law expert Deirdre Ní Fhloinn tells me. 'But the main driver of cost overruns is usually variations, often because things were started before the design was fully finished. Typically, the reason for any project being late is that those commissioning it don't know what they want. Every time something changes, it costs money and it costs time. Cranes and machinery might have to be left idle, people might have to stop working. If you're not doing the work, it suddenly costs you a fortune.'

Every construction contract has to be designed for change, she says. 'It's not like buying a car. The "product" obviously can't be seen or inspected until it is built, and multiple factors can impact on whether it is built properly, on time and on budget. The entity procuring the building doesn't always understand this. Construction contracts are like animals; they are dynamic, they have to be able to move and the price has to move with them. Otherwise, you may have to choose between stopping the project or the contractor becoming insolvent or terminating, which makes it very difficult to finish the project.'

Ní Fhloinn says the children's hospital saga shares many common features with the controversy surrounding a new Scottish parliament building. Opened in 2004, it ended up costing over £400 million sterling, compared to an initial estimate of £10–50 million. The project was delivered three years late, plagued by thousands of design changes and bad management, and grew massively in size. A public inquiry was ordered, and the resulting report criticised management of the project, including repeated underestimation of the costs involved.

'The civil servants tasked with reporting on cost estimates under-reported to their ministers. They lost control of the process, and they weren't skilled in procurement. They didn't understand how things were going to play out and where the risks were going to be. It's an incredibly complex process.'

And while those involved thought they were engaging with a contractor to deliver a piece of infrastructure, the public didn't see it this way – for them, the parliament was a symbol of Scotland.

'Similarly, the children's hospital has this enormous meaning for people that has little to do with how it gets completed and commissioned. The result is a tension, which has led to conflicts, most notably over where it should be located.'

The weight of expectation hangs over the children's hospital project at St James's, abetted by the many promises made as it was being proposed and designed. In a way, the hospital has become *Ireland's* national symbol, by which we will measure the country's success or failure. For Ní Fhloinn, this makes a public inquiry into the cost and time overruns 'almost inevitable'.

It isn't hard to see how Ireland's children's hospital fits these various analyses. The project has been 'over budget and over time, over and over again'. Instead of being adequately prepared, those building it allowed construction to begin before the design was completed. Despite mounting doubts, no one felt able to shout stop. Those who designed it went for fancy and grandiose rather than plain and functional.

The cost of building the hospital was consistently underestimated and analyses that pointed to higher expenses were suppressed. Conversely, the benefits of the hospital may have been over-represented – it will, after all, deliver very few additional beds, though they are of better quality. It could end up being under-used or it could find itself inundated with minor cases. The level of infighting between, and dysfunction in, the existing institutions does not augur well for future relations at St James's.

Optimism bias, driven by the ambition of politicians to create a career-defining monument, repeatedly contributed to unrealistic cost and time estimates. Problems such as the confined site at St James's were overlooked or made little of in the rush to win projects and create a statement building. Irish exceptionalism – this is, after all, not the first children's hospital in the world – and a failure to stand up to vested interests led to the over-speccing of the building, thereby further inflating cost and causing more delays.

These delays were so lengthy that it was almost inevitable that construction would fall victim to an external crisis. At least two of these black-swan events have occurred – an unprecedented Covid-19 pandemic and Russia's surprise invasion of Ukraine. Brexit and the 2017 Grenfell fire in London caused further shocks that impacted on the cost and design of the building; the 2026 conflict between the US and Iran may influence its running costs. At various times, these different factors have interacted, leading to even longer delays and further increased costs.

Conversely, an opportunity was missed to build in the immediate aftermath of the 2008 crash, when costs were at their lowest. In Switzerland, where I lived for a period, governments invested counter-cyclically by squirrelling away money whenever the economy was booming. In leaner times, the purse-strings would be released for major infrastructural projects in order to stimulate the economy.

In contrast, Ireland largely squandered the fruits of the Celtic Tiger. When the economic crash followed, there was little left in the kitty to cushion the blow. The construction sector was wrecked for years after, as construction companies folded and skilled staff left the country because there was no work for them.

What happened at the children's hospital was not unusual, therefore, given the experience of other countries with megaprojects. It could have been anticipated, however, and it could even have been avoided with some forethought and planning. And given how long it took the children's hospital to materialise, it is hard to understand why this didn't happen.

19

A Promise Not Kept

'We're going to make sure that by the end of this year no child waits longer in this country for a scoliosis procedure than four months.'

Minister for health Simon Harris's promise, made on RTÉ Radio in February 2017

'This is not one scandal. This is a decade in catastrophic failings.'

Parent representative Úna Keightley on the repeated spinal surgery controversies in Children's Health Ireland

Harvey Morrison Sherratt was a daredevil who did 'everything that most kids loved doing' and adored The Beatles.

Born with significant health challenges – hydrocephalus (a build-up of spinal fluid in the brain), spina bifida, scoliosis and visual impairment – Harvey was non-verbal and a wheelchair user. 'He was a big fan of going fast and doing his wheelies,' according to his mother Gillian.

At the age of one, doctors warned his parents that his lungs were being crushed by his ribcage due to the growing curvature of his spine. Scoliosis would be 'a life or death thing for him', his dad Stephen recalled the doctor saying when the couple were interviewed on *The Late Late Show* in 2025.

Scoliosis, a sideways curvature of the spine, most commonly occurs during growth spurts experienced in childhood. As well as causing pain, it can lead to a range of other health problems. Severe cases require surgery.

Because scoliosis can worsen if left untreated, time is of the essence. The longer surgery is left, the more risky it can be. Harvey was already up against the clock, but at least in February 2022, at the age of six, he was placed on the urgent surgical list at Temple Street.

That June, he ended up in intensive care with severe breathing difficulties, but his consultant said he was due for surgery in August. 'August came and went, and we heard nothing,' according to Gillian. 'In March 2023, we got a letter with a date for surgery in April, but that was very quickly cancelled without any explanation.'

As Harvey languished on the waiting list, his spine continued to curve and his health declined. That October, on social media, his mother posted an agonising video of her child struggling to breathe. Without intervention, 'he will die', Stephen warned in a newspaper interview in February 2024.

In August, when the curvature reached 110 degrees, his parents discovered he had been removed from the waiting list for unknown reasons. 'He was extremely ill, he needed regular ambulance trips, he was always in pain. It was hard as a father to watch,' Stephen said.

What really frustrates parents of children with spinal conditions, Gillian tells me, is the lack of transparency. 'You put your life on hold with a very sick child – we cancelled our wedding while waiting for surgery dates for Harvey – yet you get no information from the hospital.'

By the time he was finally operated on, on the day of the general election in November 2024, the curvature in Harvey's spine had reached 130 degrees, twice what it had been in 2022. There were complications from the operation. Some of his metal implants had to be changed out and he picked up an infection.

In July 2025, Harvey died. 'His death feels incredibly unjust,' Gillian told *The Late Late Show* two months later. 'Knowing now he was only going to live to nine, knowing that he spent the guts of three years in pain on a wait list, feels incredibly unjust. If Harvey had had timely access to healthcare, he wouldn't have missed so much of his childhood. We would have had more happy memories as a family and not so many negative memories.'

With the development board of the new children's hospital and BAM permanently at loggerheads and the public inured to stories of cost overruns and delays, the construction project at St James's had disappeared from the headlines. Sadly, children's health remained in the news, thanks to a series of crises engulfing Children's Health Ireland. Harvey's death was but one of these.

It was CHI's job to merge the three existing children's hospitals, at first organisationally and then physically at St James's. Ideally, it should have been calmly planning for the day when services were amalgamated under the roof of the new building, when it was ready. But as the completion date kept changing, CHI found itself spending more and more time fire-fighting a series of operational crises. These pointed to considerable dysfunction and mismanagement in the care of some of the sickest children in the country.

Issues with spinal surgery were nothing new in children's health. In 2008, for example, 12-year-old Ann-Marie Kelleher had to travel to Britain for an operation to correct curvature of her spine after the one in Crumlin was repeatedly cancelled. The following year, 11-year-old Jamie Murphy's surgery was cancelled due to long waiting lists and delays at the same hospital. She had to go to London twice before the life-saving surgery was carried out, funded by an anonymous donor.

That same year, Crumlin orthopaedic surgeon Pat Kiely highlighted the fact that more than 530 children were stuck on surgical waiting lists. Some of them urgently needed treatment for spinal curvature, a situation he described as 'unacceptably dangerous'.

So frustrated was Kiely about his lack of access to operating theatres to perform scoliosis surgery that with a friend he set up a charity, Straight Ahead Ireland, to do this *pro bono*. To date, it has taken 150 patients off public waiting lists.

In response to the surgeon's public complaints about a lack access to theatre time, the HSE commissioned a review of services. The resulting report was not published, but it leaked in 2011.

The report found the three Dublin children's hospitals were significantly underusing their operating theatres – Crumlin and Temple Street by 28 per cent and Tallaght by 17 per cent. It was not uncommon for theatre sessions to start late, start early, finish late or finish early, the report found, but this underuse was not due to a lack of resources or staffing.

Poor scheduling, a lack of integration between hospitals and bureaucracy were contributory factors highlighted in the report. None of the hospitals had a dedicated emergency theatre and, as a result, emergency cases were put into slots for planned operations, which affected waiting lists.

The provision of spinal surgery for children with spina bifida had been consolidated in Temple Street in 2014, though some families whose children were being treated in Crumlin chose to stay there for their care.

The problems with the service should have been consigned to the past as children's health was being reformed, but they persisted as building got underway at St James's. Once minister for health James Reilly set up the Children's Health Group (later Children's Health Ireland) in 2013, overall responsibility for spinal surgery was destined to pass from the HSE to the new body. This made sense, as spinal surgery – often urgent, complex and potentially risky – is best provided for in a unified manner in a well-equipped and well-staffed tertiary children's facility.

However, just as construction of the new hospital was taking far longer than expected, there were also delays in passing the legislation needed to set up CHI. This delayed the merging of operations in the three existing children's hospitals. The bill to create a single statutory entity for paediatric healthcare in the state didn't pass through the Oireachtas until 2018. That was, minister for health Simon Harris noted, 'an extraordinary opportunity to transform paediatric services for children in Ireland [that] will improve the experience and outcomes for children and their families'.

Finally, in January 2019, CHI formally assumed control of children's health services. The names of the hospitals changed to the awkward-sounding CHI at Crumlin and CHI at Temple Street, along with the two urgent-care centres, CHI at Tallaght and CHI at Connolly (which opened in 2019).

Unfortunately, during the hiatus that preceded this change, long-standing management and governance problems had deepened, and new ones had surfaced. And with the completion date of the new building subject to repeated postponement, the day when the staffs of the different hospitals could be joined under one roof was being pushed ever farther into the future.

Worse was to come. Discontent at spinal surgery waiting lists had continued to simmer as numbers remained high. At the end of 2016, 236 children were on the waiting list for a scoliosis operation. In February 2017, nine months into his term as minister for health, Harris made a clear promise. 'We're going to fix it. We're going to make sure that by the end of this year no child waits longer in this country for a scoliosis procedure than four months,' he told RTÉ Radio.

'That promise was well grounded. It wasn't a solo run by Harris,' says former HSE director general Tony O'Brien, who made a similar commitment at this time. 'It was grounded on a structured outsourcing plan to Germany and England, which was calibrated to remove the waiting list in its entirety – while still respecting parental choice and taking account of any special individual clinical circumstances.'

O'Brien claims the HSE-led plan was opposed by the Children's Hospital Group (later CHI) and there was 'some unease' from civil servants.

The ombudsman for children, Dr Niall Muldoon, published a report in March 2017 recognising the delays as a fundamental breach of children's rights. No child with scoliosis should have to wait for surgery more than four months, he recommended. At the time, more than 100 children had been waiting more than six months.

Muldoon described the wait times for patients in the service as unacceptable, and said young people with the condition were suffering 'severe physical and psychological effects' as a result.

The controversies in children's health continued to stack up – confounding the prospect of better outcomes for children heralded by Harris. Waiting list figures rose rather than fell in the months after the promise was made. Health managers cited delays in recruiting staff and said the four-month target could not be achieved without outsourcing up to 50 operations to other hospitals in Ireland and abroad.

The number of children waiting for spinal surgery fell in 2018 but the minister's target wasn't met. 'The record shows that the four-month target was working well but, after I left in May 2018, the appetite to push on waned,' O'Brien asserts. 'It was eventually killed under the pretext of Covid.'

With almost 50,000 children waiting to see a paediatrician for an outpatient appointment in 2019, it was clear that a solution could not wait for the completion of the new hospital.

Then came the Covid-19 pandemic. For long periods as the virus spread, people couldn't travel outside their local areas, let alone fly abroad for complex operations.

As the pandemic threat receded, the issue came back to bite the government, again and again. In November 2021, two orthopaedic surgeons from Temple Street laid bare their frustrations before the Oireachtas health committee. 'In my 20 years, I have seen the system become more and more chaotic,' Professor Damian McCormack said. 'Every little change now is the butterfly wing that is just creating more chaos. Everything is in flux. Everything is chaotic.'

'The care of children with scoliosis in this country is absolutely inadequate,' his colleague Connor Green told the politicians. 'The care of children with other orthopaedic conditions is just as bad. Therefore, the real crisis is not in scoliosis; the real crisis is everything else.'

Apologising for the long waiting times, CHI's Eilish Hardiman blamed delays on 'old and constrained' infrastructure and busy emergency departments.

The case of 11-year-old Ava Carroll, forced to wait for corrective surgery to address spina bifida for more than a year and a half, prompted Taoiseach Micheál Martin to tell CHI to 'get on with it and get it done' by tackling waiting lists for children. 'Funding is not an excuse anymore,' he told the Dáil in February 2022.

'Delays in spinal surgery have been a source of acute embarrassment for successive governments,' I wrote around this time. 'Time and again, the gruesome spectacle of young children suffering spinal deformation worsened by delays in treatment has shamed politicians into promising an end to waiting lists for young scoliosis patients.'

Promises that weren't kept but, as the taoiseach had said, money wasn't the issue anymore. In 2022, minister for health Stephen Donnelly allocated €19 million for children needing orthopaedic surgery, having been promised by CHI that the four-month target would be reached by the end of the year. The number of spinal surgeries carried out at Temple Street that year increased to 124, up from 93 in 2017.

But once again the situation got worse, not better. When spinal surgeries at Temple Street were postponed in August 2022, CHI described the move as a 'temporary pause'. Yet almost a year later, they remained paused. Though it wouldn't emerge for some time, staff had reported two serious postoperative surgical incidents. An external review of all complex surgeries on children with spina bifida was commissioned from experts from Boston Children's Hospital.

In the meantime, the ombudsman's office published another report on the service, highlighting the case of a teenage girl who was forced to wait five years for spinal fusion surgery. During that time, her spinal curvature deteriorated from 30 to more than 135 degrees.

In September 2023, the results of the Boston and another internal review were consolidated and published. An examination of the care provided by one consultant to 17 children found high complication rates, including repeated returns for surgery, and high infection rates. One of the children had died.

Connor Green, who had been so outspoken before the Oireachtas health committee two years earlier, was referred to the Medical Council and a UK expert, retired orthopaedic consultant

Professor Selvadurai Nayagam, was appointed to carry out a review. Its remit was later widened to cover all paediatric orthopaedics in the state.

The HSE confirmed that 'unauthorised devices' had been used in a small number of spinal procedures. These turned out to be non-medical grade springs inserted by the surgeon into three children.

'Things happened at Temple Street that should not have happened,' Eilish Hardiman admitted. It was 'a shocking litany of events'.

Families affected by the scandal demanded an independent statutory investigation of paediatric orthopaedics, but this was resisted. Instead, Donnelly called in the state's health watchdog, the Health Information and Quality Authority (HIQA), to review the control and oversight of surgical implants. He promised to fly in orthopaedic surgeons from overseas in a further attempt to tackle long waiting lists. He also set up a paediatric spinal task force and said he wanted hospital managers to open operating theatres for longer hours.

Meanwhile, CHI lost its chief executive when minister for health Stephen Donnelly declined to renew Eilish Hardiman's contract for a third term, invoking government policy that the chief executives of non-commercial state organisations should serve no more than two consecutive terms.

The waiting lists barely budged. Surgeons in Crumlin, Temple Street and Cappagh Hospital in Finglas were carrying out more procedures on children than before the pandemic, but this was offset by big increases in demand and referrals for spinal surgery. More than 70 children were waiting longer than four months for their surgery in July 2024. It didn't help that much of the €19 million allocated for these operations had been spent elsewhere in CHI.

Given these problems, it was perhaps not surprising that another report questioned the CHI's readiness for operating the new hospital. Top leadership were spending 80–90 per cent of their time running services in the existing three hospitals and just 10–20 per cent on the transformation into one service, according to the confidential report for the HSE by consultants KPMG, obtained by RTÉ News that September.

The report pointed to gaps in senior leadership teams, a sub-optimal clinical governance structure, a lack of clarity around the resourcing of the new hospital and the drift in expected completion dates. It also found marked differences in culture and 'organisational maturity' across the three children's hospitals.

Seven years after the promise had been made to carry out children's spinal surgeries within four months, minister for health Stephen Donnelly said he could not 'overstate the level of frustration within Government' over the lack of progress in meeting the target. It was 'unacceptable that greater progress was not made before now', he told CHI chairman Jim Browne in a letter in September 2024.

The government came under renewed pressure on the issue, with Mary Lou McDonald decrying the 'scandal' that had left children with scoliosis and spina bifida in agony and waiting years for operations. The Sinn Féin leader backed up her claims with numerous heartrending examples.

With a general election in the offing, Taoiseach Simon Harris, in a November 2024 television interview, said he accepted that he had failed to deliver on the promise he had made in 2017 but insisted that the number of children waiting more than four months had come down significantly by the time he left the Department of Health in June 2020. When he started as minister, more than 200 children were waiting more than four months for surgery and by the time he left, this figure had fallen to 35, he claimed.

Was this true? The official figures are a confusing morass of different time bands (e.g. waiting more than three months/four months, etc), operative categories (spinal fusion/spinal 'other') and dates, making it hard to make direct comparisons.

A fact check by *The Journal* found that Harris was wrong in the waiting-list figure he gave for June 2020. His party clarified that at this time, 34 children were waiting for more than three months for spinal fusion surgery not, as he had said, 35 waiting for more than four months.

Whatever about the precise figures, and the evident lack of clarity in the way they are published, the promise that no child would have to wait more than four months for surgery was not met – something the taoiseach accepted.

With crisis mounting on crisis at CHI, Donnelly sought legal advice on whether the state had powers to take over the running of children's hospital services.

One of his last acts as minister was to direct the HSE to ensure that all children waiting over four months for spinal surgery were offered the option of treatment in New York or London. It wasn't clear that this option would suit all children, given the extent of their health challenges.

The legal advice provided to the minister was that direct state intervention could take place only if an independent review identified serious failings. This wasn't long in coming, though Donnelly was soon on his way out, having lost his seat in the general election held in November 2024.

In January 2025, Lucy Nugent, the chief executive of Tallaght Hospital, became the new chief executive of CHI. The permanent position had been vacant for more than a year, since Hardiman went on medical leave. While a temporary replacement had been appointed, she left soon after to take up a new post in the private sector. After mediation, Hardiman returned to work in a new role of strategic programme director, on her existing chief executive salary.

In April, HIQA published its long-awaited report into the use of unauthorised springs in children's spinal surgeries. The use of the springs as surgical implants in operations at the hospital was wrong, according to the watchdog, while failures in controls meant that 'children were not protected from the risk of harm'.

The springs were of 'non-alloyed spring steel', which were not suitable for implantation because they corrode when in contact with moisture. They were implanted in three children between 2020 and 2022 without ethical or managerial approval or the consent of parents.

With Taoiseach Micheál Martin demanding accountability in CHI, its chairman Jim Browne resigned after 12 years in the post. Browne had told HIQA that before November 2022, the board had no sense the issues in orthopaedic surgery 'were as serious as they were later identified to be'.

HIQA's report was critical of governance structures in CHI. 'Overly complex' arrangements 'did not enable effective management and oversight of the orthopaedic service at CHI in Temple Street'. The absence of 'an open, inter-collegiate atmosphere' in the service, as well as difficulties in relationships between team members, were identified as significant contributing factors in the issues that arose.

With such overwhelming evidence of the serious failings in children's health, the government mulled subsuming CHI into the HSE.

Liz McMahon and David Ryan, the parents of Luke Ryan, one of the three children who had been implanted with an unapproved spring that later disintegrated, told reporters their son had been 'failed' by the paediatric services. 'As parents, we could never have contemplated that an experimental non-medical grade spring would without our knowledge or consent be placed in our child in an Irish hospital. Such an event was a complete breach of parental trust by CHI.' The state should step in and take direct control of paediatric care at CHI hospitals, they said.

'This is not one scandal. This is a decade in catastrophic failings,' parent representative Úna Keightley commented.

Yet the scandals kept coming. In July 2024, an independent review had been commissioned to examine if surgery carried out on children with loose hip joints – developmental dysplasia of the hip (DDH) – was necessary in all cases. It was prompted by a protected disclosure suggesting that different criteria had been used in different hospitals to determine whether the surgery was required.

In advance of publication of the audit in May 2025, CHI wrote to several thousand families of children who received hip surgery over a 15-year period and were to be offered follow-up clinics.

The audit looked at a sample of 147 hip dysplasia procedures between 2021 and 2023 at CHI hospital sites, as well as the National Orthopaedic Hospital, Cappagh.

Almost 500 children who underwent hip operations in two hospitals should be recalled for clinical review, as close to 70 per cent of surgeries had not been necessary, the audit found – 60 per cent of operations in Temple Street had been unnecessary and 79 per cent in Cappagh. In contrast, only one of the 63 surgeries examined at Crumlin hospital failed to meet the clinical criteria.

One child who received DDH surgery despite not meeting the criteria for the procedure experienced an 'adverse outcome' from the operation.

A woman whose non-verbal son received hip surgery in 2023 was among those to be told two years later that the procedure had not been necessary. 'To hear now that it was unnecessary is devastating. We trusted what we were told and why wouldn't you trust it? The guilt as a parent is overwhelming. We're supposed to protect our kids. These are real kids, and it [the surgery] has a massive impact.'

The HSE said it had already started to implement safeguards as recommended by the report, including multidisciplinary review meetings across the different hospitals and the creation of an expert panel to establish standardised criteria for the surgery. But as health journalist Priscilla Lynch asked in *The Irish Times*, 'Why weren't such safeguards already in place? Why was there no coordinated approach across the sites under CHI carrying out this surgery, given the body was created to merge the national children's hospitals before the move to the new national children's hospital?'

Further controversy ensued within days when it emerged that a CHI consultant had been reviewed in 2021 for allegedly referring public patients to his own weekend clinic. The consultant retired after the investigation highlighted issues around governance and adherence to correct procedures in a children's hospital.

The review, first reported in *The Sunday Times*, had not been sent to Department of Health officials, effectively blindsiding them and minister for health Jennifer Carroll MacNeill when it emerged.

When it did eventually make its way to the department, the report revealed an astonishing picture of the work culture in parts of one CHI hospital, where relations among some staff and between certain staff and management had deteriorated to the point that 'challenging behaviour appears to be the norm'.

A 'negative and toxic' work culture in which multiple staff complained of 'unprofessional and disruptive behaviour from consultants' contributed to the undermining of care and treatment for sick children, the report found.

Four CHI board members stepped down. In his resignation letter, Dr Gavin Lavery said the organisation had spent years challenging 'defiant' and influential hospital staff before allegations of a toxic work culture came to light. The actions of a small number, he said, were questionable and 'not in the interests of children'.

Appearing before the Oireachtas health committee in June, Lucy Nugent apologised to patients, their families and the public over 'revelations relating to our culture, governance and practices' that have led to 'great pain being inflicted upon some of those who were in our care'.

'I am sorry on behalf of the management of Children's Health Ireland and I am sorry on behalf of the entire organisation,' she said.

TDs, predictably, tore strips off Nugent and her colleagues. 'Frightening', said Sinn Féin health spokesman David Cullinane; '... absolutely zero confidence in the CHI board, zero confidence in the management,' said Fianna Fáil TD Martin Daly.

'I felt sorry for Lucy when she came in as head of CHI. She wasn't responsible for what happened before but she certainly had to carry the can,' says Paul Reid, chief executive of the HSE until 2023.

The drip drip of scandals annoyed government. After years of relative quiet, helped by unprecedented levels of investment, health scandals were, once again, dominating the agenda. Where was this leading? And, given conflicts between the HSE and CHI, who exactly was in charge of what in the health service?

'They didn't expect to be doing it for this long,' says Tony O'Brien of the 'drawn out' process of integrating the governance of the three children's hospitals. 'That has played a part in some of the breakdown in clinical governance and it has contributed to some of the problems.'

After Harvey Morrison Sherratt died in July 2025 following years on the surgical waiting list, hundreds of people gathered in Dublin city centre to remember him. They demanded an end to the suffering of children left on waiting lists for years before they could access life-changing and in some cases life-saving treatments.

Marchers carried signs and wore T-shirts calling for 'Justice for Harvey'. Honouring the wishes of the child's family, there were no political banners at the march. But opposition leaders joined his parents in calling for the resignation of Simon Harris as tánaiste.

In September 2025, Carroll MacNeill announced that CHI would be integrated into the HSE, and would cease to exist from 2027. Most of the regional paediatric units in hospitals around the country – the spokes to the central hub of the new national children's hospital – were operated by the HSE, she pointed out, so it was therefore logical to integrate CHI into HSE structures.

Carroll MacNeill agreed to set up an inquiry into spina bifida and scoliosis care in CHI, something her predecessors had resisted for some years. At the time of writing, this has yet to happen.

Some improvements were made while demand continued to increase. By the end of 2025, the wait times for a child's outpatient appointments and day-case surgery had dropped appreciably. That year, 534 spinal surgeries were carried out, but 524 patients were added to the waiting list.

Despite all the talk about sending patients abroad, only 19 children travelled internationally for procedures over the preceding two years, compared to almost 1,000 who had spinal surgeries in Ireland. Carroll MacNeill expressed 'great frustration' that this was the case, when funding was available. Acknowledging that 'not every child is fit for travel', she said there was a 'clinical element' to the low take-up of procedures overseas.

In December 2025, it was announced that Eilish Hardiman was leaving CHI for a regional role in the HSE. Hardiman had worked on the children's hospital project from 2009.

The longest-serving full-time member of staff working on the new hospital project had finally run out of road, before it was completed, a generation after it was first planned.

Simon Harris is voluble and reflective when I interview him for this book. He talks about the personal pressure he felt when the issue of soaring costs at the children's hospital hit the headlines. He acknowledges some of the mistakes that were made along the way.

There is just one issue he doesn't want to discuss. At the time we talk, in April 2026, the target of treating all children needing spinal surgery within four months still hasn't been met. Apart from confirming this fact, Harris declines to comment further on the promise he made nine years earlier.

20

No Going Back

'It did seem reasonable to me that the hospital would take four or five years to build, not ten.'
Leo Varadkar, interview with author, December 2025

'Every single date that's given is missed, every target that's set is missed. At some point, the state has to say, "Enough is enough."'
Sinn Féin health spokesman David Cullinane, May 2024

Three-time Irish Olympian, former world 5,000 metres champion and world indoor mile record-holder Eamonn Coghlan grew up a few hundred metres from the back of Crumlin hospital. 'As children, we did all our soccer and our running in the field by the rear entrance to the hospital,' he recalls to me. 'Brian [Kerr, the former Irish soccer manager] called it "the field of dreams". Sometimes, we'd even enter the hospital, looking for a chase.'

On other occasions, Coghlan had a good reason for entering the hospital – such as the day when he fractured his collarbone or was hit by a bus. 'The place was dilapidated but the care was always first-class,' he says.

After school, Coghlan went to study in the US on a sports scholarship. In 1983, at the height of his fame as an athlete, he was approached to join the American board of the Children's Medical Research Foundation (CMRF). It was to be the start of a 40-year association with the fundraising arm of the hospital in Crumlin.

An innovator in fundraising, the CMRF had become an increasingly important source of revenue for the hospital. In the early 1970s, it was raising the equivalent of €6 million a year for research, given by thousands of people all over Ireland. Coghlan's job was to develop the US side of the business. The Irish foundation was one of the first charities to raise funds through the New York City marathon. It put on 24 charity golf tournaments a year in the US. Using his athletics contacts, the world-famous athlete was able to tap rich philanthropists for donations to medical research back home.

'We went from raising two-and-a-half million punts a year to over 15 million dollars. Up to 120 runners a year came over to run the marathon in New York, and for many years they were transported with the elite athletes and given VIP access.'

The money raised was used to develop innovative techniques, such as the STING technique (Suburethral Teflon Injection, though Teflon is no longer used) to prevent urine flowing back from the bladder to the kidneys, pioneered by two doctors in Crumlin. A centre for treating children with cystic fibrosis, metabolic disorders, cancer and cardiology opened. New medical buildings in the hospital were part-funded by these charitable efforts.

Coghlan worked full-time with the foundation after returning to live in Ireland in the 1990s, and remained involved with its US board long after retiring in 2008. 'Without being crude, it was an easy sell. We were asking for money for sick children. I enjoyed every minute of it.'

With time, though, the going did get tougher. In the 2000s, it emerged that the organs of deceased children had been retained by the hospital without their parents' consent. 'Questions were being asked and we had to deal with them, but we had no idea what was going on.'

Then came the debate around the national children's hospital. 'That's when politics came into play, big-time. There were four strands to it – political, medical, academic and Church politics. But we were never brought into it.'

Initially, the government promised to raise a portion of the cost of the hospital through philanthropy. But the environment for fundraising became more difficult as the children's hospital project got delayed and the soaring cost of the project became an issue. Talk of raising funds for the new hospital was quietly shelved by CMRF in favour of existing efforts to fund research.

In 2019, the CMRF was folded into the Children's Health Foundation, which raises funds on behalf of the three children's hospitals, Crumlin, Temple Street and Tallaght. While the individual Crumlin 'brand' has been lost and staff have changed over to new structures, Coghlan is not given to pessimism about the future.

Fundraising will inevitably be important for the new hospital after it opens. The way to sell it to donors is to spread the message about the creation of a new centre of excellence, he says. 'Americans love positive messages. We just have to tell them how great it is.'

Even the delay in completing the new hospital doesn't faze him. Crumlin and Tallaght hospitals both took 20 years to build after they were proposed, he points out.

What should happen to the old hospital buildings in Crumlin, beside his childhood 'field of dreams'?

'The work done by the many volunteers who raised millions and millions over the years for Crumlin should be acknowledged. If the site is sold, the money should go straight into CHI, to be utilised for what we originally fundraised.'

The timeline had slipped, but at least now, in 2023, there was an agreed date of October 2024 for completing construction. The building was said by the development board to be 90 per cent complete, though David Gunning, its chief officer, warned that the last 10 per cent is often 'the slowest to complete'. Allowing time to commission the building, children would surely be attending the hospital as patients in 2025.

Or would they?

Appearing once again before the public accounts committee, Gunning admitted it was a 'possibility' that the hospital would not open until early 2026. 'I think the optimism has been beaten out of all of us in relation to this project,' he told TDs in October 2023.

By the end of 2023, the approved budget of €1.433 billion had been used up. Even so, the Department of Health sought a pay increase for the latest incumbent to chair the development board.

Fiona Ross, the chairwoman of the National Library and a former stockbroker, had been appointed back in September 2021, eight months after Fred Barry had left.

By January 2024, Donnelly too was doubting the previously announced completion date. The development board was sceptical of the completion dates put forward by the contractor due to continuous delays, he said.

Back in 2016, then minister for health Leo Varadkar had promised that the hospital would be up and running by 2020, 'short of an asteroid hitting the planet'.

'At the time I said that, there was nothing coming to me, either on paper or verbally, that this date could be way off,' he tells me.

Was the comment over the top?

'It was certainly wrong. It was what I honestly believed. It did seem reasonable to me that the hospital would take four or five years to build, not ten.'

In 2024, with the building still unfinished after eight years, it fell to Varadkar as taoiseach and his fellow ministers to bow to the inevitable. The budget allotted to the project was increased to €2.24 billion.

This was the 'maximum allocation' and no further funds would be provided, Varadkar insisted. He predicted 'years of disputes' with the contractor, even after the hospital opened.

The news that government was allocating so much extra to the project came as no surprise. 'For years now, the question has not been whether the budget for the hospital will exceed €2 billion, but by how much,' I wrote. 'That question was dodged as part of a deliberate strategy to ensure there would be no going back at the point when the bad news ultimately emerged.

'The new "final" figure of €2.24 billion makes the striking building under construction at St James's Hospital in Dublin one of the most expensive hospital builds in the world. Despite multiple assurances from ministers, there is no guarantee the final cost will not be even higher.'

After all, I added, 'why should anyone believe anything about a project that was supposed to cost €250 million, then €450 million, then €750 million, then €1.4 billion and then €1.7 billion, before reaching its current stratospheric level?'

In another era, this kind of overspending would have sparked severe cuts, probably bringing down a government. Back in 1982, a Fine Gael/Labour coalition fell after proposing a tax on children's shoes and an additional two pence on the price of a pint. Roll on 40 years, and the government planned to shell out an additional €500 million and more on an already profligate project, yet few even blinked an eye.

Why? Because the state was awash with cash.

As during the Celtic Tiger years, the Irish economy was once again the envy of Europe. Total annual tax take had reached almost €110 billion. A surplus of more than €8 billion was expected at the end of 2024. Engorged from strong growth in the economy and a boom in corporate tax payments, the public finances could take the hit from the cost overrun at St James's.

What a numbed public cared about now was when the hospital

would open. It was clear that this wouldn't happen in advance of the next general election. But at least ministers on the campaign stump could point to progress, in the form of a building just off the South Circular Road that was, allegedly, on the point of accepting patients. For the politicians, it was fortuitous that the hospital wasn't yet open. If it was, there would inevitably be teething problems, generating negative headlines. As it was, the issues of delays and overspending were off the front pages. I and other journalists had found other, more productive health stories to write about.

Up at St James's, the cranes were finally gone, the external façade was complete and the first of 100,000 pieces of specialist equipment was being installed. But a further delay in completion was signalled in May 2024.

The deadline for completion of the building had slipped back to February 2025, with patients unlikely to be admitted before August that year.

Tánaiste Micheál Martin rounded on BAM, accusing the contractor of failing to resource the project sufficiently 'for quite some time'. The deadlines it set were 'likely to be part of a commercial strategy ... to try and extract more money and funding from the Irish people', he claimed in the Dáil.

BAM issued its habitual rejection of these claims, denying that the project was under-resourced and claiming design changes ordered by the development board were the primary reason for delay.

Just days after his cabinet colleague had attacked the company in the Dáil, Taoiseach Simon Harris and other government ministers attended a ceremony in County Louth marking the start of work on the €100 million Narrow Water Bridge. The contractor for the project was BAM.

At the end of May, development board officials appeared once again at the public accounts committee. About 1,600 claims for additional payments made by BAM were subject to the dispute management process, TDs were told, but so far the net change to the contract value from adjudicated claims was just €27 million, less than 3 per cent of the original contract value.

What the board representatives failed to mention was that BAM had just been awarded an additional €107 million under the independent conciliation process set up to resolve disputes.

Donnelly had been made aware of the award but the official answering TDs' questions was not briefed on it until after the meeting. The development board's reasoning was that the conciliator's recommendation remained confidential as it could still be appealed to the High Court.

The board rejected the conciliator's findings, and another recommendation that the formal completion date for the hospital – before any potential penalties could apply – be extended by more than a year. Under the mechanisms in place, BAM was forced to start High Court proceedings in order to access the additional payment, and to guarantee that the money would be repaid if it lost the case.

BAM had by then made 2,311 claims with a total value of

€793 million. Eighteen individual claims accounted for the bulk of this sum.

The board claimed BAM had committed to deploying up to 1,700 workers on the site, but never actually engaged more than 1,260. In 2024, the average number of workers was 811, it said. The contractor, though, insisted it had adequate resources in place.

As the months passed, further problems arose. Some 1,200 smoke detectors and 400 fire exit signs needed to be moved 'to ensure compliance', according to the board. It expressed concern about the quality of construction work in parts of the hospital; BAM rejected these claims. Just one firm remained in the tender process for operating the parking at the new hospital, a less than ideal situation. The board notified BAM of its intention to seek liquidated damages of over €21 million for late completion. The completion date looked like it would slip again.

The board claimed BAM was offering up rooms as completed when they weren't. The building contractor described the issues as minor and routine – 'nothing a quick run of the vacuum cleaner wouldn't fix', a BAM source claimed to me.

In September 2024, the completion date set by BAM slipped back four months, to June 2025 – the fourteenth time this deadline had changed. Construction of the hospital was 31 months behind schedule. And as the delay grew, so did the amount being claimed by the contractor.

Simon Harris, who was minister for health when the clearly problematic contracts with BAM for phase A (below ground) were signed in August 2017 and phase B (above ground) in December 2018, was now taoiseach.

It was 'absolutely right and proper' that the board was standing up to BAM, Harris told reporters in the US in September 2024, where he was attending United Nations meetings.

'This is the source of all the problems that have beset the building of the hospital – weak contracts that don't protect the public purse, don't hold the developer to delivery dates and don't allow for effective oversight of the project,' Sinn Féin leader Mary Lou McDonald reminded the Dáil in the taoiseach's absence.

Even at this late stage, not a single room in the hospital had been completed to the satisfaction of the development board. 'There are 5,678 clinical spaces in the new hospital, and whilst, to date, BAM has offered 3,128 as complete, none were completed to the required standard,' Gunning told the public accounts committee in September 2024. 'We are averaging about 13 to 15 defects per room. These aren't scuffs of paint. These are compliance issues,' project director Phelim Devine said.

The handover of rooms and de-snagging of minor issues was 'a process, not a one-off event', BAM responded. 'Rooms are never presented as final until the completed building is handed over to the customer.' More than 1,500 new drawings had been received in 2024 alone, with new ones continuing to arrive on a daily basis, the company complained.

It singled out changes to the ceiling plans that required BAM to revisit the vast majority of ceilings. More than 2,200 smoke detectors, sprinkler heads and other ceiling-mounted devices had to be removed and reinstalled.

In the committee meeting, David Gunning robustly disagreed: 'Design is not holding up the project at the moment. These rooms are partially finished.'

With no one believing the hospital would be completed as promised by June 2025, Donnelly met senior executives of Royal BAM, the Dutch parent company of BAM Ireland. He came away with a commitment by the contractor to complete by that date but still felt that 'given deadlines have come and gone we would all be naive to come away and think that's sorted'.

'My view and the view of our board is that they simply have not had enough workers on-site. There ... haven't been enough people on-site finishing off this hospital.'

A general election was called in November 2024. The public accounts committee sought to call witnesses from the development board and CHI once again before the campaign started, but they were unavailable. The alternative dates they proposed were during the election campaign, when the committee couldn't sit. Overspending at the St James's site receded into the background as other issues took centre stage.

One brief exception arose during a televised leaders' debate, when the moderator, journalist Katie Hannon, said Harris had 'personally signed the contract that brought us the children's hospital saga' when he was minister for health.

Harris interrupted to say, 'Well of course I didn't.' Hannon pointed out that as minister for health he was ultimately responsible for the contract. 'The government of Ireland made a decision to build the National Children's Hospital and I was a part of the government,' he added.

The taoiseach spent the days that followed insisting that he was not seeking to dodge responsibility for the overspend at the hospital. While he was technically correct, he admitted to having been 'unnecessarily pedantic and semantic', he told reporters while on the campaign trail.

'The buck stops with me,' he said, speaking on Newstalk FM. 'The point I was trying to make is [that] there's sometimes comments that are a little flippant, like one person signed off on the contract.

'These things go through a very deliberative process. Lots of departments look at them; lots of bean counters in different departments. There's a board, [the] National Paediatric Hospital Development Board, and then the minister of the day, in this case me, would bring a proposal to cabinet rather than sign a contract.'

Though Fine Gael trailed in third in the election after Fianna Fáil and Sinn Féin, Harris clung on to power with a continuation of the rotating taoiseach arrangement with Micheál Martin. Stephen Donnelly lost his seat.

In December 2024, an updated programme of building works for the hospital was agreed, for the first time in almost four years.

With both sides working towards the June 2025 finish date, an end seemed to be in sight. But with the operational commissioning of the building now expected to take at least six months, a new problem loomed. According to the Department of Health, migration to the hospital could not happen in winter due to 'clinical risks'. Its opening would be delayed once again, to 2026.

Early access to the site for CHI was supposed to begin in April 2025, but was delayed because many areas were deemed not to have been completed to the contractual standard.

The deadlines slipped for a fifteenth time. Substantial completion was delayed until September 2025, with the first patient intake not expected until June 2026 at the earliest. The board put it down to a reduction in staffing by BAM; the builder said the project was 'fully resourced'.

Ironically, the first part of the project to be handed over, in December 2025, was the Ronald McDonald House accommodation block for parents, connected to the hospital by an underground tunnel and built by a different contractor.

It wasn't hard to see a loss of nerve in the decision announced in June 2025 to name the new institution the National Children's Hospital Ireland. Following the Phoenix hospital debacle, the planned facility had remained nameless, despite a grassroots campaign to have it named after Dr Kathleen Lynn. Eight years after the botched effort to name the building after a mythological bird, ministers approved the most basic name available to them.

The name, preferred over 16 other options, was picked because it reflected 'the vision of the new hospital being a hub in a national network of paediatric care'. A 'simple and straightforward' name was needed, minister for health Jennifer Carroll MacNeill said, so worried parents would end up exactly where they wanted to go, regardless of potential language barriers.

The minister then entered into a public spat with BAM, just as her predecessors had. Accusing the company of failing to employ enough staff on-site, she claimed in August 2025 that BAM was not drawing down the maximum funding available to get the hospital ready for the September deadline.

BAM issued a statement expressing disappointment at the minister's remarks, and claiming large areas of the hospital had been finished since early July and offered to the board. Carroll MacNeill issued another statement the same evening, describing BAM's account as 'not credible'. Less than 15 per cent of rooms were satisfactory and these were 'chequer-boarded' throughout the building rather than being concentrated in a single zone that could be accessed early.

And so the arguments continued in circular form, the two sides repeating their mantras, leaving the public none the wiser as to where the truth lay, or when the hospital would open.

STATUS OF DISPUTES BETWEEN BAM AND THE DEVELOPMENT BOARD, AS OF 25 MARCH 2026

- Number of claims notified by BAM: 3,505
- Number of these claims substantiated by BAM: 3,388
- Value of substantiated claims: €899.6 million
- Number of substantiated claims on which the employer's representative has made a determination: 3,141
- Total value of these claims by BAM: €806.19 million
- Value of these claims determined by employer's representative in favour of BAM: €53.16 million
- Percentage of determinations in favour of BAM against total value claimed: 6.6 per cent
- Number of determined claims (3,141) challenged by BAM: 2,619
- Value of these claims being challenged: €1,067.34 million
- Number of these disputed claims with a value of less than €10,000: 1,980
- Total value of these smaller disputed claims: €2.55 million
- Total value of biggest disputed claims: €926 million, for 18 claims for extension of time
- Percentage of overall claim value represented by these 18 claims: 87 per cent
- Increase in contract sum up to 25 March 2026 due to employer's representative determinations, agreed conciliations and adjudications: €60.23 million
- Increase in contract sum as a proportion of contract value: 6.6 per cent
- Additional amount paid to BAM for construction inflation: €48.75 million

- Number of sets of High Court proceedings involving BAM and the development board: 5
- Liquidated damages development board will seek, based on BAM's forecasted completion date of 30 April 2026: €40.2 million
- Development board's estimate of the sum at dispute, when allegedly duplicate claims are removed: over €300 million
- Sum that development board believes BAM is entitled to claim: €0

21

What Went Wrong?

'It's one of the greatest buildings in Ireland. But is it what we needed?'

Paediatrician Jonathan Hourihane, interview with author, January 2026

'I think errors were made at the start.'

Leo Varadkar, interview with author, December 2025

Anyone who passes through Dublin 8 regularly is probably familiar with the imposing new building that has materialised at the back of St James's Hospital. Approaching it from the South Circular Road, the children's hospital glows warmly above the surrounding red bricks, the lights on its upper floors seemingly forever on.

Driving by the building on one of 2026's hot summer evenings, I thought back to something Mary Harney had said more than 20 years ago. At the time, her party, the Progressive Democrats (PDs), wanted to sanction a string of privately run hospitals on public land. The party's stated aim was to provide much-needed hospital beds at a lower cost than building them publicly.

Addressing her party conference in April 2005, Harney made the point that 'hospitals are very expensive to build and equip, and they could absorb every last euro available'.

The PDs' proposal met with suspicion and significant opposition, and eventually collapsed. None of the proposed private facilities – including one proposed for the land later used for the children's hospital – was built. And Harney rowed in behind the ill-fated plan to build a public children's hospital at the Mater.

The party's failed attempt to privatise part of the health service seemed like a fork in the road. Thereafter, public investment was prioritised. State spending on health has tripled since 2005. Yes, the population has increased and aged, and provision has improved in some areas, but the service doesn't feel three times better.

And yet the first half of Harney's prediction has come true. The children's hospital has proved very expensive to build and equip, much more than anyone imagined. If it hasn't emptied the coffers, that is only because the state has been lucky in recent years and is awash with cash.

Is there an iron law that says health projects are bound to be phenomenally expensive, I wondered, and, moreover, prone to big delays and cost overruns? Or were the problems at this children's hospital avoidable? The result of mistakes made along the way?

As the record shows, lots did go wrong here. The errors were multiple, compounding their impact. Delay built on delay; overrun on overrun. The more serious the mistakes made, the harder it became to undo them, or even to avoid repeating them. People who are digging a hole and find something has gone wrong invariably keep digging (which is, literally, what happened here). The longer the project continued, the greater the potential impact of external events. And this is even before the challenge of operating the hospital has been met.

Let's consider the main reasons the building of this hospital has been so delayed, and has involved such enormous expense.

LOCATION, LOCATION, LOCATION

Children's hospitals around the world get built in nearly every type of location. Some are downtown; others lie on the periphery of cities. Some buildings reach for the skies in crowded urban locations; others are spread out, low-slung, surrounded by parkland. Ireland's version could have been built on a variety of site types and still have been made to work.

As contributors to this book have made clear, there is a philosophical divide over the optimum surroundings for such a hospital. Some experts say fresh air and green fields are important and even have a therapeutic value. Others say the children attending tertiary hospitals are often so sick that they don't care if their room offers mountain views or a playground outside; they just want to get well, obtain the best treatment and have their parents close by.

Ireland's new children's hospital admirably attempts to bridge this divide by providing cutting-edge medicine *and* generous recreation facilities, notwithstanding the hospital's location near Dublin's city centre on an already crowded hospital campus. When I lived in Dublin 8, around the time the hospital was first mooted, there wasn't a single football pitch in the postcode area. The children's hospital adds four acres of gardens and open space planted with 400 trees, albeit for the use of patients, staff and visitors. The 'rainbow garden' alone, one of Europe's largest rooftop gardens, is the length of Croke Park.

There is a price to pay for this, given the cramped location. Building at St James's has added hugely to the cost of the project. The Dolphin review put the premium for building on a brownfield site (previously developed land) at 25 per cent compared to a greenfield location. A second report also found there was an additional cost, which it estimated at 5 per cent a year — or a cumulative increase of two-thirds in the decade the hospital has been under construction. Neither report attracted much attention nor changed what happened.

Twice, the national children's hospital was designed for tight urban spaces. The Mater site was challenging, with little room for parking, and surrounded by historic buildings and narrow streets. St James's had similar issues; site preparation took far longer than originally anticipated. Anxious to proceed with the project as quickly as possible, politicians overlooked the impact of conditions at the chosen location. Because space was limited, gardens, a pool and a helipad had to be provided on upper levels, adding significantly to the cost.

St James's made sense on medical grounds, and it has good public transport links. And, remember, building on a greenfield site such as Blanchardstown wouldn't have been as cheap as was claimed. 'If we had had lots of money, Blanchardstown might have been an option,' James Reilly says. 'If you were going to go with a 20-year plan to build adult and maternity hospitals. But think of the money that would have cost. And at a time when the Troika was in town.'

Reilly says that, when he was minister for health, the debate was all about the location of the hospital. 'Costs became an issue well after I left. There were no costings that you could rely on at that time.'

At the time it was chosen, I thought St James's was a good location. I knew many leading hospitals around the world had been built in city centres – why should Ireland do things differently? The land was available for free. The adult hospital there has top-class facilities, and I hoped building the children's hospital in this often-overlooked part of Dublin could help drive a regeneration of the area and further improvements in public transport.

These are considerable advantages, but they have to be set against the challenges of the site. Now, I realise that many of us misunderstood the contribution location made to the increased cost of the hospital, when this was magnified by other pressures and delays.

START LOW, FINISH HIGH

Many different amounts have been cited for the cost of this hospital. At the Mater, it began with an official price tag of €500 million and, later, €650 million. It is difficult to know how realistic these figures were. An internal letter from 2008, not published at the time, refers to the project costing between €800 million and €1 billion. One early member of the development board tells me that, by 2010, after close scrutiny of the plans, his assessment was that building the hospital was 'maybe achievable' for €1–1.5 billion. 'These projects are extremely difficult [to cost],' he points out. 'There are so many moving parts to them.'

So the bill for the project, for which no cost–benefit analysis was ever published, was underestimated long before it moved to St James's. Where there was talk of money at this time, it centred on the wasted outlay at the Mater, though that seems like small beer now.

Lowballing – low initial estimates of cost – moved up a gear when the project moved to the new location. In its application to build the hospital, St James's estimated 'total construction costs' for the building at just €297 million. Adding design fees, VAT and other items, the overall estimate was €484 million. Four years had passed, and yet the projected cost of the hospital being built in a new location was estimated to be the same as at the Mater, or even lower.

St James's committed to building the hospital 'within the SJH campus' by 2015, a mere three years later. With 'very limited' decanting requirements, access to the site would be possible, it claimed, in under six months. All of this was fantasy planning, as later events would show.

Politicians and officials would have paid little heed to the back-of-an-envelope calculations made by St James's and other hospitals, according to a number of sources interviewed for this book. Yet the public did, not knowing any better.

Lowballing wins public acceptance for a project, while misleading people about how much money is actually needed. The result is the swallowing up of public funds that might have been more productively spent on other projects. And, when the truth emerges, the public feels it has been taken for a fool.

Underestimation continued after construction began. For several years, the official estimated cost of the children's hospital project stayed stubbornly at €650 million, despite increasing inflation and setbacks. It remained so even as internal analysis, which wasn't published, was suggesting a price tag of up to €1 billion.

Within that estimate, the provision for risk and inflation was 'nonsense', a highly placed source admits. 'If a pharmaceutical company had as little definition to the project as we had at that stage, they'd have added 40 to 50 per cent to the estimate. But if we had given the real cost, we'd have been told, "Don't build it!"'

When building design was completed and costs started to soar, officials were slow to give ministers the full details, and ministers were just as tardy about telling the voters. In the end, those running the project simply stopped estimating the cost in public.

'Should we have done things differently? Absolutely not,' one of those centrally involved in the project says. 'Were we always honest about costs? No!'

Artificially low estimates of the cost of building the hospital in the early stages helped secure approval of the project but stored up trouble for later on, when the real cost became evident. Construction went ahead, but the subsequent controversy was inevitable, given the gap between public expectation on price and the reality on-site.

In late 2018, the government was forced to acknowledge that the project now needed funding of €1.43 billion. This figure was a stop-gap, as the issues that had pushed up costs to that point had not gone away. However, it remained the quoted figure for four years.

Since early 2024, we have been told that the project will cost €2.24 billion, and not a penny more – here's hoping past performance does not predict future results.

HUBRIS AND OVERELABORATION

The national children's hospital is the largest enclosed building ever constructed in Ireland. It is also the country's biggest hospital. Its design and inner workings are complex, because it is a facility for very sick children.

'Hospitals are complicated. They're not like hotels,' according to a senior figure involved in overseeing the project. 'They provide intensive care around the clock. They have a large number of beds and employ thousands of staff. And it's not just about the kids; you have parents going through perhaps the most traumatic experience in their lives.'

That leads to uncertainty around design and budgeting, he says. 'That's been our experience in Ireland, and it's the experience of every other country that has tried to build something different.'

Ireland has built thousands of kilometres of motorway, and hundreds of schools and primary-care centres, but these smaller projects are predictable in their design, and therefore replicable. In contrast, the new hospital is big, unique, bespoke.

Everyone agrees on the complexity of the hospital; there is no consensus on whether the level of design was right. 'The scale of the project was a function of medical politics – everybody working there wanting their own rooms,' this individual continues. 'That was let slip. It should never have been allowed to escalate the way it was. It needed better leadership and control.'

It is striking how prominently design issues featured throughout this saga, from the oversized building planned for the Mater site to the statement architecture at St James's. Much could be justified by saying it was needed 'for the children of Ireland'.

'Everyone involved wanted an iconic building – the paediatric community, consultants, the Department of Health, the HSE,' one civil servant observes.

'There's too much hospital in this by a mile,' is the opinion of Brian Gilroy, the former HSE executive who went on to build numerous nursing homes and other health facilities in the private sector. 'It's over-briefed. There's something for everyone in the audience.'

Members of the development board from the hospital's early phase insist the plans for the hospital were closely scrutinised to ensure value for money. Yet John Gallagher, the businessman who briefly chaired the board in 2010–11, didn't feel the project had enough staff at the time to ensure full cost and scope control.

'It's an impressive building. It looks phenomenal. It's one of the greatest buildings in Ireland,' says paediatrician Jonathan Hourihane of the later version of the hospital designed for the St James's site. 'But is it what we needed? Massive medical and architectural hubris built something like that.' Hourihane's view is that the location is correct but 'the wrong hospital' has been built there. 'It's too elaborate, too fancy. It could have been built cheaper and smaller, but on the St James's site.'

An engineer closely involved in building the hospital summarised for me two of the main concerns expressed about its design: 'It is crazy to have single rooms for all patients. And the curves didn't help.'

The decision not to accommodate any children in wards was made early. Most children's hospitals in the US are single-occupancy rooms. The UK and Australia tend to have a mix of largely single rooms with some multi-bed rooms. Internationally, the direction of travel in hospital design in this century has been towards exclusively single rooms, even before the Covid-19 pandemic. In this respect, the hospital at St James's *is* following international best practice.

'You don't win a contract to build a big children's hospital unless you offer something sexy,' according to Eoin O'Morain, former chairman of Scott Tallon Walker Architects, which designed a children's cancer hospital in London but was unsuccessful in bidding for the Irish project. 'But extra spec adds to cost. So many of the rooms are curved – can you think of anything more expensive? You don't have to have the best, you need something that works.'

Brian Gilroy is another critic of 'curvy, bendy' design: similar to Professor Björn Flyvbjerg, he believes public projects such as hospitals should be built straightforwardly, 'the same as with Lego blocks: you put down a few blocks, then another few on top of the first ones, and so on'.

Not everyone agrees: John Martin, the planner who spent over five years on the development board, believes the extra cost came not from over-design but from 'the scale and complexity of a medical building' and changes made to the original design: 'I don't think the design was a huge cost factor – not even the curved walls.'

Why not aim high, some say. 'We had one chance at this, building the best children's hospital in the European Union,' a doctor tells me. 'It's going to be there for the next hundred years. I think cutting costs on that would have been foolhardy.'

The building at St James's, with its spectacular glass and aluminium roof and multi-floor atrium, is born of a desire to create what the French call a *grand projet*. This is a monumental hospital that will be used by families from across the island of Ireland for decades to come.

There was a sense of it being 'payback time' for all the years of hardship and poverty the country has experienced; remember that for years it was hoped the project would be ready for the centenary of the 1916 Rising. By the time the real cost became evident, though, it was too late to make savings.

Perhaps less might have been more, once the basics were in place. The building being 'iconic' or winning architectural awards was 'never an issue of interest to the politicians', according to Leo Varadkar. Sinn Féin's David Cullinane believes the hospital should have been designed simply: 'no bells, no whistles, no frills'.

Varadkar adds: 'I doubt any politician would ever say, "Build me a curved hospital that costs more and takes longer to build." If anyone had ever come to me with a decision between a curved building and a rectangle, I would have told them to build a rectangle – and put a nice tower beside it, like a hospital in an American city.'

Even then, costs could have been controlled by specifying the brief in detail, and sticking to it. Yet the project grew over time – for example, the number of day beds more than doubled despite a declining birth rate.

Given the complexity of modern hospitals, those developing them have two options, O'Morain says: 'Build a generic hospital building, don't consult with the users, and tweak it when the doctors arrive; or design it with the stakeholders, agree the number of beds and theatres and everything else, but don't change anything afterwards.

'At St James's, they tried to consult with people as they were going along. The surgeons were saying they needed bigger, better theatres. So you ended up with many changes. You can't procure a hospital with these kinds of tender methods.'

But critiques of the hospital tend to vary according to the underlying philosophy of the person making them. For some, the play areas and hanging gardens in the building are mere frippery, distractions almost from the business of getting well. For others, the child-centred environment of the new hospital isn't just pleasant, it will help young patients heal.

'This idea that you have to have areas where children can look at trees and grass, it sounds nice,' says Karl Anderson, the parent of a child treated at Crumlin who went on to become a communications adviser to Brendan Drumm in the HSE. 'But when you're sick, you're sick. If you're well enough to enjoy these features, you need to be going home, to be treated by your local clinician.'

'This hospital is all about the child,' a paediatrician tells me, setting out the therapeutic argument for the design. 'It has curves because that's what children love. It was built around the patient; it's like going into Disneyland. And that's a form of wellbeing, a form of healing.'

High cost wasn't just the result of elaborate design; it also had to do with the many changes made to the original plans. BAM, for instance, claimed in September 2024 that it had received over 23,000 revised design drawings from the development board in the previous five years.

Many of these changes were minor, but some were big – hundreds of tons of extra steel in the roof, for example. 'Certain people, two years or three years down the road after agreeing what the layout was, were saying, "No, we want plugs over here and we want this facility to have this entrance", or whatever,' says someone who was closely involved in designing the layout of the building. 'Once you start doing that, the price escalates.

'I remember sitting in meetings with some of these docs and stopping the meeting and calling people out and saying, "Don't treat us like this." It was like somebody getting a box of Meccano at Christmas and wanting another box because there wasn't enough in the first one. The message that once you lock things down you don't reopen them didn't get across to some clinicians who were coming back to have things redesigned. The hardest word you'll learn in building something like this is the word "no".'

The new hospital will be a landmark in Dublin for most of this century. It is right that the hospital has been planned to the highest standards seen in other countries, for instance by providing single-bed rooms for patients. It is right, too, that there was ambition around the design of such an important civic building. But it is hard to see where proper account was taken of the cost of using statement architecture and the finest construction materials, particularly in the awkward site that was chosen. And it is also hard to understand why so many changes were made as the building was being designed.

The result is a building that was more expensive to build, and one that is likely to be expensive to operate.

SPLITTING THE 'G'

'G' here stands for governance; at the children's hospital, it was complicated. Brendan Drumm, Tony O'Brien and others attribute many of the project's problems to the decision by minister for health James Reilly to split the functions of the National Paediatric Hospital Development Board (NPHDB) between two bodies. The board had been around since 2007, when it was created to build and then operate the hospital. In 2013, by decree of the minister, it was reconstituted to become responsible solely for building the hospital (the so-called 'build board'). Operational responsibilities passed to the Children's Hospital Group, later Children's Health Ireland (CHI).

The build board certainly benefited from the expertise of the professionals appointed to it – builders, lawyers and other specialists with considerable construction experience. There were limits to their expertise, though. None had dealt with a project of this size and complexity before, and most had more experience in the private sector than the public one.

Prior to 2013, the development board was required to make

judgement calls on requests from doctors and others for facilities in the new hospital, and to deal directly with the cost implications of any alterations. 'This is a critical governance issue for all hospital developments, where the demands for space and facilities by clinicians are understandably often way beyond what can be financially justified. A balance has to be achieved,' Drumm says.

After the decision was made to separate the running of the three existing hospitals from the building of the new one, 'you had a governance structure where an operational board could request significant changes in the design or expansion of the hospital without being responsible for the additional construction costs. Meanwhile, the development board charged with building the hospital within budget had no opportunity to interrogate or challenge the clinical or operational justification for the changes'.

'This governance structure was always going to result in massive cost overruns,' according to Drumm. 'And this is what happened, with the contractors having to deal with thousands of requests for alterations in the design as the building progressed.'

Mary Harney, a predecessor of Reilly in the Department of Health, also believes it was a mistake to split the building and operational functions between two bodies. 'You had the development board in charge of the hospital and this other crowd coming in saying, "We need this, we need that, we need the other." It's crazy. It's no wonder it's gone the way it has.'

Leo Varadkar put through the legislation to repurpose the build board. 'The view at the time was that the budget and project was too big for HSE Estates while still doing all their other work. A dedicated statutory body was needed,' he says.

'In relation to infrastructure, a lot of people argue that you need a bespoke body or bespoke legislation or both for really big projects. This was an example where we had a bespoke body in charge of construction and I'm not sure it was so great. HSE Estates did a pretty good job with capital projects, so I wonder would we have been better off giving it to them. Who knows? But that [splitting the board functions] is what we did.'

Frank Dolphin says that when the decision was made to advance the project by turning the National Paediatric Hospital Development Board (NPHDB) into a 'build board' filled with construction experts, he recommended to the minister and his officials the creation of an interim group to liaise between the development board and CHI. This didn't happen. 'I knew that it would take a lot of managing – you have 200 paediatric consultants there with strong views. A structure was needed to control and integrate these, not to mention the opinions of others – nurses, physios, occupational therapists, porters.'

Tony O'Brien is adamant the splitting of the original board had a 'critical' impact on the project and was the most important factor affecting later costs.

'Before the HSE was established, the department had within it a hospital planning office – engineers, quantity surveyors, a big team that occupied half a floor in Hawkins House. They were very effective managers of building projects, most of which came in on time, on budget. They were very good at value engineering, which is a nice way of saying cutting the costs of a project in order to get the whole thing that you want.'

When the HSE was established in 2005, this expertise was transferred into it, as part of a bigger estates function within the new organisation. 'The department no longer had any of that capability, just a few people managing the capital financial side. The HSE, therefore, had all that expertise. But at the point at which this decision was made, the HSE was due for abolition.' (Ultimately, it survived.)

James Reilly, a trenchant critic of the HSE when in opposition, did not want it in charge of the children's hospital project, and neither did some of his fellow ministers. The result, O'Brien says, was the new incarnation of the development board, repopulated with limited HSE involvement and a direct line into the department.

'So you had this three-legged stool – the HSE was the funder, the [development] board bore all the responsibility for developing, designing, procuring and eventually handing over the finished product, and the Department of Health was responsible for supervising all that,' O'Brien explains.

'But it had no hospital building expertise left within it. That was all over with the HSE, to one side from the central role. Consequently, there were lots of mixed messages. We were telling our people, "Keep control over this, make sure that they have sensible plans, that the procurement is right." On the other hand, politicians in the department were telling them to "build a flagship hospital, make it spectacular".

'When you have people questioning, as they do now, the impact of the shape and physical form of the hospital or the cost – semicircular walls, for example – it's very clear that that was driven by the desire to build a flagship hospital. Value engineering would never have allowed that. But the department didn't have any value engineering capability left in it.

'Tom Costello was a great guy, I have a lot of respect for him. But the board was taking instructions from the political system as to what they were to build. A political system that was supported by a department that had no expertise within it, to match the board's. It was not a balanced governance process. They went off and did what they were told to do. It's a fantastic-looking building but very expensive.'

The project would have benefited from greater capacity or expertise within the Department of Health, Simon Harris acknowledges. 'It did strike me during my time as minister for health there wasn't a capital buildings unit in the department, because it had all been outsourced from the HSE. Therefore, they were very reliant on the advice from the HSE and the Department of Public Expenditure, and expertise available to the government. With the benefit of hindsight, that wasn't robust enough.'

Reilly says his governance reforms were motivated by a desire to avoid the infighting he had witnessed years earlier as a GP during previous hospital mergers. He wanted the build board to get on with constructing a huge, highly technical hospital while CHI focused on bringing together the professionals who would work in it.

The development board included the head of procurement in the Department of Public Expenditure to monitor the budget, he points out, while HSE Estates was represented on CHI. But the hospital had become more complex by the time it reached the planning stage, he observes.

The creation of the build board did have one fortuitous consequence for government ministers – it could be endlessly blamed for the delays and cost overruns that occurred, even though many of these problems were rooted in decisions made elsewhere.

THE TWO-PHASE CONTRACT

It wasn't just governance that was split in this project; in 2017, a decision was taken to progress construction in two, connected phases. In the first, the contractor would dig the hole for foundations and, in the second, the seven-storey building with its 6,000 rooms would be constructed. The design of the building was to be finalised while phase one was ongoing, thereby allowing work to begin early and saving time overall. However, without a final design, the price could not be known until much later.

'The procurement was a mess of a decision,' according to Professor Paul Davis of Dublin City University's Faculty of Business. 'Effectively, they were writing a blank cheque.'

The two-stage approach isn't inherently flawed, he says, but for it to work, the design must be sufficiently mature and the transfer of risk 'real and contractually enforceable'. Neither condition was met at St James's.

'I don't know why anyone thought it was a good idea. It seems like a strange way to go about things,' Leo Varadkar says of the two-phase arrangement.

The main reason it was adopted was to save time. 'If we had gone for the one-stage contract, it would have taken years and years before we could have gone to tender,' says John Martin. 'We would have had to progress the design to a much fuller stage. The two-stage option seemed to us a way of getting started, while building in time to make refinements.'

Government and the development board were also afraid the complexity of the project would put off potential bidders. There weren't many players in the Irish market capable of taking on the job. A number of large contractors decided not to bid, sources say, thinking the challenge was too risky to undertake. The two-stage process was a way of attracting builders into the project without feeling they were over-committed at that early stage.

A lack of bidders wasn't the only concern. What if the company building the hospital collapsed? Around this time, concerns were being raised about Carillion, the UK's second largest construction company. It ultimately went into liquidation in 2018 with debts of over €7 billion and 2,000 job losses. A subsequent inquiry blamed the British government for outsourcing contracts based on the lowest price. The national children's hospital could not be allowed to fail in the same way.

At St James's, the two-phase arrangement meant a contractor would be awarded the tender before the detailed design was completed. However, this also meant that the contractor was legally entitled to make claims at a later stage. And this is what happened. Further, while some amount of inflation proofing was included in the contract, it proved insufficient as the economy boomed.

'The design was still evolving while the contractor was being appointed and pricing was being fixed,' Paul Davis says. As a design develops, the basis for pricing shifts: 'Where the contractor is pricing against a design that is not stable, and which changes significantly thereafter, the state retains substantial risk, whether intended or not. That creates prolonged negotiation rather than clean transfer.'

'Everybody thought the guaranteed maximum price that was agreed was based on a detailed design, but it wasn't,' according to one of those close to the process. 'The amounts of materials required weren't properly represented. So when BAM was finally approved to start the second stage, and the detail was more complete, the price had gone up to €1.43 billion.'

Under the two-phase arrangement, significant risk in the project shifted from the contractor to the development board. The government had little alternative but to adopt it, this source claims, because building firms were loath to take on phase one: preparing the site in such a cramped location. 'The view from the procurement people was that we wouldn't have got people to bid because it's too complicated. We had to de-risk the site first.'

Remembering back to one of my visits to the site, these points about its complexity seemed to make sense. On the first occasion, I saw the many buildings that had to be cleared, and heard about the services that had to be moved elsewhere, and the big underground sewer that would have to be moved. On the second occasion, the buildings and the sewer were gone, and there was a huge hole in the ground, deeper than any I had seen before, there or elsewhere. Vast curtains of concrete reinforced the sides of the hole, dwarfing the local houses perched above this enormous crater. I was no civil-engineering expert, but I could see that this wasn't straightforward work.

It didn't help that, effectively, the contract was awarded on price alone. 'It goes back to who else was going to build the hospital,' says Simon Harris. 'We were very limited in our options. This is a problem to this day in this country – attracting in good people to deliver projects.'

The two-phase method had been used before, in motorway design. 'This contract came utterly recommended,' says one supporter of this approach to procurement. 'BAM were invested from the start. There was a partnership approach and a familiarity with the larger project.'

So while the approach wasn't entirely novel, made the project more attractive to potential bidders and promised to save time, it left those commissioning the hospital exposed on price. 'Competition left the marketplace once the preferred bidder was selected,' Paul Davis says, leaving the state negotiating with one supplier for phase two rather than competing in a live marketplace. 'Ultimately, they looked for the cheapest and they got the dearest.'

As Orla Hegarty of UCD's School of Architecture has pointed out, procurement is about balancing the project requirements and money available against prices in the market, quality control and the management of risks. The objective has to be good value for money, rather than low prices, as well as a means of comeback for defects.

Davis says the contract with BAM lacked adequate levers to hold the contractor to account if it failed to deliver. Procurement is not simply about running a tender, he says; it is about how those commissioning a job manage the supplier relationship over the life of the contract. When the competition for the tender ended, these levers were the only remaining control mechanisms for the board.

The state should have negotiated harder to put these levers in place and ensure it carried less of the risk, he argues. Under the contract drawn up with BAM, the only levers the board had were to refer disputes to the employer's representative, impose liquidated damages, or terminate the contract. The first two had little impact on the dispute that arose, while the third was unrealistic because of the delay it would cause.

'The state has allowed the marketplace to dictate what is done, instead of dictating to the marketplace,' Davis says. 'If it can't manage the market, every infrastructural project will end up in a similar scenario. At the end of the day, the state did not manage BAM. But how, you would have to ask, could a private contractor not be managed by the might and breadth of the state? It's not about the development board, it's about the state.'

So the two-phase contract, while not new, was an unusual and potentially risky approach. Its use did avert the danger of the builder collapsing during the job, which would have been a disastrous outcome. This approach promised a quicker delivery, but it is not apparent that this happened.

When a contractor was chosen for the first phase, there was little option but to continue with the same contractor in the second phase of building the actual hospital. The risks to the state could have been minimised by negotiating a contract that included levers to hold the contractor to account where problems arose, but this did not happen. Overall, it's my view that the two-phase contract was poorly chosen and badly executed.

A LOVELESS MARRIAGE

The much-publicised row between the NPHDB and BAM Ireland blew up long after many of the other problems with the hospital. The dispute might never have occurred if the earlier flaws around location, governance, costs, design and procurement had been avoided or rectified.

In summary, BAM blames delays and rising costs on design changes made by the NPHDB after construction started, while the development board alleges over-claiming, under-resourcing and poor execution by its main contractor. As of July 2026, BAM is suing the development board for about €1 billion in additional claims while the development board is seeking €40 million in liquidated damages.

Deciding who is right in this quarrel is difficult. The minutes of meetings of the development board are published with heavy redactions. BAM communicates with the public by press release. While the issues at the hospital are reviewed regularly by Oireachtas committees, the level of scrutiny exercised in these forums is largely superficial and the TDs asking the questions lack technical expertise. Ultimately, the commercial court will decide the issues between the two sides.

How much did the development board itself contribute to the problems with BAM? Feeling it had no other choice, it ran a tender process skewed towards price, and this produced an inevitable result. BAM won the contract for the children's hospital with a tender that was €131 million less than the closest bidder. Members of the development board who were in the room when the bids were opened recall the sharp intake of breath that occurred when it became clear that BAM had won. But they can hardly have been surprised.

Long before the children's hospital project, the company had a reputation for bidding low for public contracts. Arguably, it can bid lower than rival firms by drawing on the resources of a parent group in the Netherlands. But it also had a reputation for 'extracting maximum value from contracts', as one architect puts it, through subsequent claims. But even BAM may not have anticipated the soaring inflation and staff shortages that occurred after it had submitted its bid, and which threatened to erode its profit margin. 'BAM priced at the bottom of the market and everyone has been paying for it since,' according to one official who oversaw the national children's hospital project for many years.

As BAM began work, the claims started coming in. Initially, relations were civil, with the development board's experienced personnel believing they could manage the company's hard-nosed stance, as had happened on other big projects. A dispute-resolution mechanism had been set up and was working.

At this time, management on both sides comprised construction-industry veterans who were well versed in the shifting relations and tough bargaining seen on many building jobs. 'You cannot deliver projects without relationships,' an industry insider points out. 'You can have all the contracts and guaranteed maximum prices in the world, but if relations break down, your projects will fail.'

Conditions change on all building jobs as they progress, and with them the final cost. At St James's, problems arose over delays in completing a design for the hospital. Where a full design is completed before building starts, the scope for additional claims is limited. But at the children's hospital, there was no full design, so changes were inevitable – and so were further claims.

Reports point to incomplete design as the main early cause of cost overruns. As the PwC report found in 2019, the vast majority of the €450 million increase in the budget was due to an underestimation of what it would cost to build the hospital. Far less derived from claims by BAM and other contractors. And even then, the cost of mechanical and electrical systems at the hospital was rising faster than the cost of building it.

Cost pressures worsened as inflation soared and external events, such as Brexit, caused problems. With the hospital seriously over its (underestimated) budget, cost was bound to become the subject of political controversy.

Relationships soured as these issues went public. From here on, government (and opposition) politicians focused their ire on BAM, availing of legal privilege to make claims in the Dáil or at Oireachtas committees. The company took umbrage, and relations on-site worsened. The lead officials at the development board left, and a new, more combative leadership was installed. BAM Ireland's senior management also changed after long-time chief executive Theo Cullinane retired in 2022, with managers from Royal BAM's English subsidiary drafted in to front the company's Irish operations. The new executives on both sides were less familiar with their opposite numbers and less inclined to meet them halfway.

Despite talk of thousands of claims, the dispute between the two sides centres on a small number – just over 20 – involving large sums of money. The aggregate claim sum is also misleading, as it derives from adding all of the individual claims, though many are overlapping. To give an example, the list of claims might specify a requirement to move five sockets in a room, with each socket listed separately, when in reality this work will be done by one person on the same occasion, at a smaller global cost.

Many people I have talked to feel there is a basis to BAM's assertions about changes in design, but that the impact of these have been exaggerated. 'There could be an element of truth to all that [the claims],' one senior civil servant concedes, 'but it doesn't explain the full story.'

'BAM should have been finished three years ago,' says a board member who does admit to a 'grudging respect' for the company before it became the butt of political attacks. 'They can whinge and moan all they like, but it's not that different a hospital today than was originally conceived. All complex medical and pharmaceutical projects change along the way.'

The company is entitled to have its claims adjudicated through the conciliation machinery set up for the project and to take court proceedings if it remains unsatisfied with the outcome of conciliation. Its scope to do this would have been limited if the development board had drawn up a contract with sufficient leverage to rein in contractors.

BAM has won awards of over €140 million from the conciliator, Ciarán Fahy (who died in September 2025), and time extensions of 300 days. In Fahy's view, the company's claims clearly had some merit. The board disputes these awards and seems to be betting heavily on a more favourable outcome in the commercial court.

Was BAM big enough to be able to resource the project properly? Would any Irish contractor have been able to allocate sufficient resources at a time of widespread staff shortages in key areas? Perhaps, a formal joint-venture might have provided more options.

Notwithstanding the problems at the children's hospital, BAM has prospered in Ireland in recent years. And, despite all the rancour at St James's, the company continues to build bridges, roads, colleges and other projects for the state, without any visible fuss.

NOVELTY, LUCK AND CIRCUMSTANCE

A lack of prior experience was evident in the management of the project from the very start. Tallaght was the last new hospital built in Dublin, almost 30 years previously and only one-third of the size. The children's hospital was a bespoke project, a one-off of a scale and complexity that had never been seen in Ireland before. There wasn't a playbook to repeat, its governance was flawed and the small group of staff running the project were permanently stretched. As *Irish Times* journalist Pat Leahy commented: 'There's a strong sense that lots of people were making it up as they went along. So nobody really knew how to get to grips with cost control.'

The project sat awkwardly at the interface of the public and private sectors. 'The way things were set up, it was like getting boys to do men's work,' says someone from a private-industry background who was closely involved with the project in the early days at St James's. 'You set up a board but restrict pay, so the best people don't apply. You don't allow enough people on the board to be able to run a massive project. And you don't separate the design and management of the project.'

'I think the errors were made at the start,' Leo Varadkar says. 'Once it was going to James's, once you did the two-stage thing, once BAM got the contract, what sort of project management from anyone would have made it much better?'

The location of a single hospital was always going to be contested, given how many competing interests were affected. But opposition mushroomed as the project failed to communicate a vision. For years, it has been pushing into a headwind, in part due to this failure to communicate. Despite spending heavily on public relations, those behind the project too often stayed silent in the face of criticism favouring different approaches or locations for the hospital. All kinds of claims were made about other options without being rebutted, resulting in a public that was sceptical about the project even before the controversy about costs blew up.

The involvement of a slew of government agencies didn't seem to improve the quality of decision-making. The children's hospital wasn't a Department of Health solo run, insists Simon Harris. 'Nobody ran into government with a piece of paper on this – the departments of public expenditure, health and finance, and the HSE, they were all involved.'

People operated in good faith and there is no reason to doubt their bona fides, he says. 'It's easy to say "terrible health" or "terrible minister X or Y", grand. But it highlights a more fundamental issue around expertise on capital projects within government.'

Bad luck played a role. The idea of a single national children's hospital was given the go-ahead and a site chosen, in 2006, in the Celtic Tiger era. The economic crash hit immediately after that. Building costs halved between 2007 and 2010, but the hospital was still on the drawing board, not ready to begin construction. Years were then lost to arguments and the failed planning application at the Mater. Construction costs remained depressed when tendering took place at the new location at St James's, but, by the time the project really got going, Ireland was booming again. Construction coincided with an extended period of hyperinflation, Covid-induced interruptions and supply chain issues.

If building had gone ahead as originally planned in 2011, it might have been started cheaply. The government would have supported the construction sector when it most needed help, in the aftermath of the crash. Even so, the Mercer's Institute for Successful Ageing, a seven-storey building like the children's hospital (though only a fraction of its size), was built at St James's between 2014 and 2016 for under €50 million. The contractor was BAM.

The children's hospital, of course, was a megaproject, something so large it altered the economy in which it was located. By sucking in all available resources – and more – it created its own price environment. As I've written, the problems of such projects are by no means unique to it, or to Ireland. Megaprojects of this kind have run into turbulence in other countries. But there are ways of minimising the challenges they face.

In the early 1960s, British prime minister Harold Macmillan was asked what had most blown his government off-course. He replied, 'Events, my dear boy, events.'

The modern version of this is 'stuff happens'. The children's hospital project was buffeted by Brexit, the Covid-19 pandemic, the Ukraine war and, as the building was nearing completion, the Iran conflict. All of these external events added to cost and contributed to delays. Individually, they could not have been foreseen, yet something – some unpredictable event – with the potential to knock the project off course was always bound to occur. Designing in detail and constructing at speed is one way of dealing with such a risk, but the opposite happened at St James's.

22

'This must never happen again'

CHI finally got access to the new hospital – or, more precisely, to a single floor of it – in December 2025. Cleaners were despatched to the sixth floor with its 360 rooms in advance of the planned installation of equipment.

Even this small step forward came eight months later than scheduled. 'I wish BAM would just give me the hospital,' Jennifer Carroll MacNeill said the following month. When would it be finished? 'I'd love to tell you,' the minister for health lamented to journalists.

By late March 2026, the hospital was projected to be 40 months late, compared to the original contract date. The total cost incurred by the development board for a still incomplete hospital was €1.644 billion. People stopped talking about completion deadlines after they were missed for the nineteenth time. The board was now complaining about dust in ventilation ducts and 106,500 room defects; BAM complained about the use of 'highly selective data' about the state of the project.

The building once set to be named after a phoenix became an albatross around the neck of seven successive ministers for health.

The development board has gone through eight chairpersons since it was set up. The idea of a single national children's hospital that was proposed in 1993 and approved by government in 2005 is slowly becoming a reality in 2026. Building it has taken ten years since the granting of planning permission and nine years since formal sanction, about twice what was envisaged.

The hospital didn't use up 'every last euro available', as Mary Harney predicted, but that was only because governments were flush with income. As it was under construction, the tax take from multinationals mushroomed to the extent that a week's Exchequer receipts would cover the entire cost. In Leo Varadkar's words, 'the hospital was always a "hundreds of millions problem" rather than a "billions problem" like Brexit or tax policy.'

It didn't bring down the government either, though there were a number of tight no-confidence votes. Essentially, Brexit came along to distract people.

The project has been a bruising experience for many, amid the rows and resignations. 'People got an awful drumming at times,' one of those involved in its planning tells me. One witness who appeared before the public accounts committee describes it thus: 'I was 57 going into the meeting. And I felt like 97 coming out of it.'

Still, Simon Harris, the minister who came under most fire, survived to become Taoiseach. The hospital's chief architect, Benedict Zucchi, now chairs his firm, BDP. The development board is still employing staff long after it might have expected to have completed its work. In 2025, BAM's Irish subsidiary paid a €53 million dividend to its parent company in the Netherlands.

Through its budgetary failings, the children's hospital sucked up funds that might have been used for other health projects. It also destroyed confidence in Ireland's ability to plan major infrastructure. The last new public transport project, the Luas Cross City, was completed in 2017. Dublin's massive MetroLink project has been in planning for more than a decade, but it remains unclear how much it will cost ot when it will be finished. The latest estimate is €19 billion, twice what it was four years ago. More than €525 million has already been spent and construction is yet to begin.

But the children's hospital is there now, the best in the world, according to Zucchi. It is an idea become reality that has to be made to work, a building that has to become a functioning service for children. Staff from different institutions with different traditions have to be brought together successfully. Governance failings within CHI need to be fixed. The new institution has to work purposefully with St James's and the HSE. It has to be run affordably, and within budget. Soon enough, a maternity hospital will be needed in order to achieve the trilocation of hospitals that the experts say provides the best care for mothers, babies and children. With birth rates falling, the quickest solution might be to fold a maternity unit into the existing building.

'I think it will be great when it opens, just like T2 in Dublin Airport, the Port Tunnel or the Luas – all projects beset by construction delays and overruns but which are greatly valued today,' says Varadkar. He points to infamous examples of cost overruns in other countries – such as Berlin's new airport, delivered €5 billion over budget and nine years late. Big projects are hard to do in democracies, quickly and on budget, is his point. 'In many countries in the world, the most expensive building is an air-force base or a palace or a mosque. In Ireland, it's going to be our children's hospital. That's a good thing – even if it doesn't justify the project taking ten years and costing whatever it's going to cost.'

Perhaps he's right – and Harry Crosbie too, when he says: 'At the end of the day, we're going to have a world-class hospital. Five years after it has opened, no one will care about the cost.' After all, everyone who has seen the new building so far loves it.

Must we always get wise after the event, though? And forget so quickly? On a rough tot, the children's hospital is a minimum €1.3 billion over the original budget (even if this was an underestimate). About 5,000 social homes could have been built with that, or more than 1,500 hospital beds. Depending on what happens in the courts, the final overrun could be worse. And with the hospital being completed almost a generation late, something like 900,000 children have missed out on the chance of being treated in it.

Yet the workings of the project haven't been properly scrutinised since the PwC report back in 2019. Its operations remain largely opaque. A circular row between the development board and BAM drags on, while very little attention is paid to other aspects, such as the performance of the design team and of other major contractors.

In Germany, a public inquiry was held into the Berlin Airport fiasco. Scotland conducted a public inquiry into overspending (by a factor of ten) on its parliament building. What would an equivalent Irish inquiry into the children's hospital find? How can we contemplate not holding one, given what has happened? And how can we embark on other major infrastructural projects without properly learning from the mistakes made on this one? (Already, the projected cost of the new National Maternity Hospital is about 13 times the original estimate.)

Despite the talk of lessons learned, we know overspending continues to dog public projects. In the past few years, the Arts Council wasted €7 million on a failed computer system, while the Office of Public Works was criticised for spending €1.4 million for a security hut and €336,000 for a bicycle shelter.

Yet these botched undertakings are minuscule compared to the outlay and overspend on the children's hospital. I am reminded of the words of Linda Dillon, one of the campaigning parents from Crumlin: 'This must never happen again, in any area of life, especially where services to the public are involved.'

We have come a long way as an independent nation. In 1919, Dr Kathleen Lynn founded St Ultan's hospital with £70 in the bank and two cots in a room. Over a century later, the national children's hospital will open with almost 480 beds and an operating budget likely to exceed €1 billion a year.

What Lynn lacked financially, she made up for through hard work and a personal connection with her patients, and by making her hospital a centre for medical innovation, based on the best new approaches she learned in other countries.

The new children's hospital and its staff could do worse than to follow her example.

Timeline

1969: A report recommends that Temple Street children's hospital should be 'closely associated' with the Mater hospital nearby. This proposal is not acted on and the hospital's management continues to develop services on the existing site.

1972: A study group recommends that paediatric services should be consolidated in two hospitals in Dublin, one on each side of the Liffey.

1981: The Department of Health pushes for the National Children's Hospital (NCH) on Harcourt Street to join the Meath and Adelaide adult hospitals in moving to the new Tallaght Hospital, while guaranteeing its role as a teaching hospital for Trinity College.

1984: The department announces a plan to construct a new hospital to replace the existing buildings on Temple Street. Nothing happens due to health-service cutbacks.

1989: The government decides to upgrade Temple Street by relocating it to the nearby Mater Hospital. Within a few years, problems arise, with concerns over planning and financial implications leading to uncertainty about the development.

1993: Plans to merge the three Dublin children's hospitals – Our Lady's in Crumlin, the NCH and Temple Street – on the site of an adult hospital are proposed by the Faculty of Paediatrics of the Royal College of Physicians of Ireland. The recommendation is ignored by successive governments, who feel that upgrading the three facilities separately is a better idea.

Temple Street opens discussions with the Mater about transferring to the Mater site.

1998: The NCH closes its doors on Harcourt Street and moves to the new Tallaght Hospital.

1999: A €300 million plan is unveiled for a new children's hospital for the northside of Dublin, to be located on the site of the Mater. The announcement is made by Taoiseach Bertie Ahern, local TD for Dublin Central, and then minister for health Brian Cowen. The new facility will replace Temple Street.

2001: The government promises a national review of paediatric hospital services. Plans are unveiled for the move of Temple Street to the Mater and the upgrading of buildings at the Mater.

2002: Parents set up the New Crumlin Hospital Group to campaign for the redevelopment of Our Lady's Hospital. In December, they publish the Pollock report, in which a UK expert recommends that the building be replaced.

2003: Dublin planners give the go-ahead for the six-storey children's hospital planned at the Mater.

2004: The Progressive Democrats (PD) leader, Mary Harney, succeeds Micheál Martin of Fianna Fáil as minister for health following a government reshuffle.

2005 January: The Health Service Executive (HSE) is created as the single provider of public health and social care services in hospitals and communities nationwide.

2005 April: Harney, speaking at the PD annual conference, says the replacement of Crumlin hospital is a priority for her.

2005 June: Professor Brendan Drumm, a paediatric gastro-enterologist at Crumlin hospital, is named as chief executive of the HSE.

2005 August: Drumm takes up the post. Harney puts the plan to move Temple Street to the Mater on hold.

2005 September: Harney initiates the review of tertiary paediatric hospital services promised four years earlier. She says Crumlin should be replaced at another site.

Drumm, addressing the Oireachtas committee on health and children, says the national paediatric hospital 'should ideally be in the city centre or close to the Mater site'.

2005 December: The HSE commissions the long-promised review of tertiary paediatric hospital services from international consultants McKinsey & Co.

2006 February: The *Children's Health First* report by McKinsey recommends a single tertiary children's hospital in Dublin that is easy to access, has space for future expansion and is colocated with an adult hospital with academic facilities.

The actual site for the hospital will be chosen by a task group made up of officials from the Department of Health, HSE and the Office of Public Works.

2006 June: The task group picks the Mater campus as the site of the hospital and this is endorsed by government. There are many objections by interest groups to the site.

2007 March: The government appoints businessman Philip Lynch to chair the National Paediatric Hospital Development Board (NPHDB), which will oversee the project.

2007 May: Members of the NPHDB are appointed.

The selection of the Mater is opposed by both Tallaght and Crumlin. Questions about the selection process are raised in the Dáil. Harney defends the choice, citing its central location and ability to bring about the quick delivery of the project. Private developers offer to build the hospital at no cost to the state, on a greenfield site near the M50 motorway.

2007 October: The HSE publishes a framework brief for the hospital prepared by consultants RKW.

2009: Taoiseach Brian Cowen, announcing the appointment of architects for the project, says the hospital will be open by late 2014.

Crumlin agrees to take up its seat on the development board.

2010 July: Prominent medical commentator Dr Maurice Neligan criticises the choice of the Mater as the site for the hospital.

2010 October: Lynch is sacked by Harney due to 'significant and fundamental differences' with the minister over the choice of the Mater. Harney says it is not in the remit of the board to 'revisit the government decision taken on the location of the new hospital'. He is replaced by another businessman, John Gallagher, but the controversy continues.

2011 January: Harney tenders her resignation as minister for health.

2011 March: James Reilly of Fine Gael is appointed minister for health following a general election.

Gallagher resigns as chairman of the NPHDB after five months, saying he is at 'risk of incurring further material ongoing costs in the project without full government support'.

Lynch says the decision to locate the hospital at the Mater was 'a political decision, a northside job', an allegation the HSE and Harney deny.

2011 May: Reilly announces another review into the decision to build at the Mater, to be conducted by international experts.

2011 July: Reilly receives the report of the review affirming that the correct site was chosen for the children's hospital and reaffirming the principle of colocation with an adult hospital. A planning application is submitted.

2011 October: An Bord Pleanála oral hearing into the project opens.

2011 November: Reilly pledges the new hospital will open in 2016.

2012 February: An Bord Pleanála refuses permission to build, saying the proposed development would 'constitute overdevelopment'. It says the height, scale and form of the proposed facility means it will have 'a profound negative impact on the appearance and visual amenity of the city skyline'. The government is forced back to the drawing board, six years after it was first decided to locate the national children's hospital at the Mater. A new site will have to be found.

Another review group is established, led by businessman Dr Frank Dolphin. It considers six adult hospitals in Dublin: a revised project at the Mater, Beaumont, St James's, Tallaght, Connolly Hospital in Blanchardstown, as well as a proposal from the Coombe maternity hospital.

2012 June: The Dolphin review group reaffirms the colocation principle and identifies St James's Hospital as a suitable site. The site is seen as advantageous because the hospital already has teaching facilities, 'excellent' public transport access and is close to the Coombe. But the review group also warns that the construction of new children's and maternity hospitals on the site will stretch the site's capacity, and that it will be more expensive than building on a greenfield site.

Two of the Dolphin group's members, planners Simon Clear and John Martin, carry out a further assessment of the planning implications for each location.

2012 November: The government announces that the project will be built on the campus of St James's Hospital, on a larger site than originally envisaged by the hospital.

More delays follow and the St James's site attracts criticisms similar to those levelled at the Mater, many of which are to do with its location in the city. Opponents say the site is too small, with poor car access.

The project is promised for 2016.

2013 August: The NPHDB is established by statutory instrument, now with the core responsibility of building the hospital. Merging the existing hospitals and operating the new one will be the responsibility of Children's Hospital Group, later Children's Health Ireland (CHI).

2014: The design team of architects, design engineers and quantity surveyors is appointed.

2015 April: The design for the new hospital is unveiled.

2015 August: Minister for health Leo Varadkar announces a planning application for the €650 million development is being lodged, with the project slated for completion by 2020 if permission is granted. Procurement for the enabling works on the site begins.

2016 April: Planning permission is granted after a three-week oral hearing. The hospital will have 380 inpatient rooms and 93 day beds, and 1,000 parking spaces for families and staff. The hospital will be supported by satellite clinics in Tallaght and Blanchardstown.

Varadkar says the hospital will open by 2020 'short of an asteroid hitting the planet'.

2016 June: The tender process begins. The contract for the enabling works to clear the site is awarded to BAM Ireland, one of the state's largest building firms. A two-phase approach to procurement is adopted.

2016 August: Enabling works begin at St James's. As opposition continues, an opinion poll finds 73 per cent of people believe St James's is the wrong site.

2017 February: BAM is awarded the contract to build the foundations, basement and hospital itself.

2017 April: The government gives the go-ahead for building the hospital and two satellite centres, based on a 'definitive business case' pricing the build at €983 million. Minister for health Simon Harris says the hospital will open in 2021.

2017 June: A fire in Grenfell Tower in London kills 72 people and prompts a review of fire regulations in tall buildings internationally. Dublin City Council demands the installation of sprinklers throughout the children's hospital, a decision confirmed later by An Bord Pleanála.

Leo Varadkar is appointed taoiseach, succeeding Enda Kenny.

2017 August: BAM signs the main works contract. The NPHDB is told costs have risen by €200 million.

2017 October: The government and CHI announce the name of the facility will be Phoenix Children's Hospital Ireland.

2017 December: The European Investment Bank undertakes to provide a €490 million loan for the construction of the hospital and two urgent-care centres.

2018 March: Detailed design of hospital is completed.

2018 April: The naming proposal is withdrawn after hefty criticism and legal threat from the Phoenix Children's Hospital in Arizona in the US. By then, the CHI had spent over €40,000 on the naming plan.

BAM submit further cost claims totalling €200 million.

2018 June: John Pollock, project director of the hospital, warns HSE and Department of Health officials of 'cost challenges and pressures' affecting the project. He blames construction inflation, 'gaps' in the design and 'resistance' to meaningful engagement by the contractors for the problems arising.

2018 August: The project team tells the board of an estimated €191 million cost overrun. Harris is made aware of the potential overrun, but later says that he didn't know the exact figure and asked officials to investigate what the final cost would be.

2018 November: Harris is told the project is €450 million over budget.

2018 December: Taoiseach Leo Varadkar tells the Dáil that the project will now cost €1.433 billion. Several other capital health projects may have to be delayed due to the overspend, he says.

The completion date is now August 2022.

2019 January: BAM starts main works on the hospital building.

Two Oireachtas committees conduct investigations into overspending on the project and consultancy firm PwC is commissioned to review the cost escalation.

2019 February: Tom Costello, chairman of the development board, resigns. He is replaced in April by Fred Barry, former head of the National Roads Authority.

Varadkar, speaking in the Dáil, accuses 'some companies' of lowballing contracts. BAM issues a statement calling on the taoiseach to clarify his 'inappropriate and damaging' remarks.

2019 March: The project director for the hospital, John Pollock, tenders his resignation.

2019 April: PwC finds a 'series of weaknesses' involving initial planning, budget oversight and execution of the project. Most of the €450 million overrun since 2017 was down to an underestimation of the initial costs, it says. There were 'significant failures' in planning and budgeting, and all but €16 million of the overrun could have been controlled.

2019 July: The urgent-care centre in Blanchardstown opens.

2019 September: David Gunning, a former chief executive of Coillte, is appointed chief officer of the development board.

2020 March: The construction site at St James's is forced to close due to the Covid-19 pandemic. It remains closed for 14 weeks. BAM submits a revised programme, pushing back the date of substantial completion.

2020 April: The board begins legal proceedings against BAM.

2020 November: Gunning accuses BAM of not committing enough resources to the project; this is denied by the contractor.

2021 January: Fred Barry steps down after two years chairing the development board. He is succeeded in July by Fiona Ross, a former stockbroker.

2021 April: BAM sues the development board over outstanding claims.

2021 November: The urgent-care centre in Tallaght opens.

2022 February: Russia invades Ukraine. Increased energy prices add to the cost overruns on the hospital project.

2023 July: Varadkar says the €1.43 billion budget for the hospital will have to be increased.

2023 October: The board announces the date for 'substantial completion' as 29 October 2024, more than two years late.

2024 February: The government allocates maximum funding of €2.24 billion for the project. This figure makes it one of the most expensive hospitals in the world.

The Dáil public accounts committee hears of further delays to the completion of the hospital. The development board blames the delays on lack of resourcing by BAM. BAM blames design changes demanded by the board's design team.

2025 May: Tánaiste Micheál Martin tells the Dáil that BAM 'has not resourced this project sufficiently for quite some time'. Days later, government ministers attend a ceremony marking the start of work on a €100-million bridge in County Louth, to be built by BAM.

The completion date is put back to September – the fifteenth time in over four years that a promised completion date has not been met. Patients are unlikely to be admitted until mid-2026.

2025 December: CHI gets access to the sixth floor of the hospital.

2026 April: The date of substantial completion of the project is delayed for the nineteenth time. The hospital is unlikely to open until 2027, possibly in the second half of the year.

Bibliography

BOOKS

Ahern, Bertie, *The Autobiography*, Arrow Books, 2010

Barrington, Ruth, *Health, Medicine & Politics in Ireland 1900–1970*, Institute of Public Administration, 1987

Browne, Noël, *Against the Tide*, Gill Books, 1986

Collins, Stephen, *The Power Game: Fianna Fáil since Lemass*, The O'Brien Press, 2000

Drumm, Brendan, *The Challenge of Change: Putting Patients before Providers*, Orpen Press, 2011

Earner-Byrne, Lindsey, *Mother and Child: Maternity and Child Welfare in Dublin, 1920s–1960s*, Manchester University Press, 2007

Flyvbjerg, Bent & Gardner, Dan, *How Big Things Get Done: The Surprising Factors Behind Every Successful Project, from Home Renovations to Space Exploration*, Macmillan Business, 2024

Gilmore, Eamon, *Inside the Room: The Untold Story of Ireland's Crisis Government*, Merrion Press, 2016

Hanna, Michael, *The National Children's Hospital of Dublin: A Social and Institutional History 1822–1998*, A&A Farmar, 2022

Kennerk, Barry, *Temple Street Children's Hospital: An Illustrated History*, New Island Books, 2014

MacLellan, Anne & Mauger, Alice (editors), *Growing Pains: Childhood Illness in Ireland, 1750–1950*, Irish Academic Press, 2013

McAuliffe, Mary & Wheelock, Harriet, *The Diaries of Kathleen Lynn: A Life Revealed Through Personal Writing*, UCD Press, 2023

Shovlin, Phil, 'A Strategic Decision-Making Process – An Evaluation', MScMgt thesis submitted to Trinity College Dublin, March 2007

Tussing, A. Dale, *Irish Medical Care Resources: An Economic Analysis*, Paper 126, Economic and Social Research Institute, November 1985

Varadkar, Leo, *Speaking My Mind*, Sandycove, 2025

REPORTS

Report of the Consultative Council on the General Hospital Services, chaired by Professor Patrick Fitzgerald, Department of Health, 1968

Recommendations for Dublin Paediatric Services, Faculty of Paediatrics of the Royal College of Physicians of Ireland, 1993

Pollock, Dr Ronnie, *Analysis of Facilities Provision at Our Lady's Hospital for Sick Children, Crumlin, Dublin 12*, 2002

Report of the Panel Reviewing the Events Surrounding the Death of Roisin Ruddle, Department of Health and Children, 2005

Children's Health First, McKinsey & Company, 2006

Report to the Minister, Review Group on the National Children's Hospital, chaired by Dr Frank Dolphin, 2012

National Paediatric Hospital Development Board: Report on Preliminary Observations in Relation to the Construction Capital Cost Escalation of the National Children's Hospital, Mazars, 2018

New Children's Hospital: Independent Review of Escalation in Costs, PwC, 2019

Acknowledgements

This book was written between autumn 2025 and summer 2026, as the construction of the national children's hospital at St James's trudged to a long-delayed conclusion and preparations could finally be made for its opening.

I interviewed dozens of people whose paths crossed with the national children's hospital project over its lengthy period of gestation and execution. Those who were happy to be quoted are referenced in the text; others preferred to speak off the record. I am extremely grateful to all of you.

In addition, I would like to thank the following who provided background information about the history of children's health in Ireland, particularly since the 1990s: the Royal College of Physicians of Ireland; Professor Brendan Drumm; Professor Chris Fitzpatrick.

The Tyrone Guthrie Centre in Annaghmakerrig, County Monaghan, accommodated me for a week of blissful quiet when I was working on a late draft of this book. I am very grateful for the centre's hospitality.

I have the good fortune to have Jonathan Williams, as my agent, to carefully shepherd my scribblings towards the printed page.

My thanks go also to my editors at Hachette Ireland, Ciara Considine and Joanna Smyth, for their careful handling of this text.

Some of this book was written in the reading room of Rathmines Library, a Carnegie institution I have haunted since I was a small boy. Long may it prosper.

Paul Cullen

August 2026

pcullenmedia@gmail.com

www.ingramcontent.com/pod-product-compliance
Lightning Source LLC
LaVergne TN
LVHW040534240926
848761LV00038B/365
9781399755894